Meal Planning Strategies, Tips & Techniques

Meal Planning Strategies, Tips & Techniques

A Practical Handbook For Everyone

Written By:
Kristine Sinner, MS, RDN, CEDRD

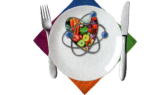

Edited & Designed By:
Jessica Garvar, WiseMindMarketing.com

Copyright © 2019 by Kristine Sinner, MS, RDN, CEDRD

All Rights Reserved

Except as indicated in the Limited Duplication License below, no part of this handbook may be reproduced, translated, stored in a retrieval system, or transmitted, in any form or by any means, electronic, mechanical, photocopying, microfilming, recording, or otherwise, without written permission from the author.

Although the author and editor have made every effort to ensure that the information in this book is correct, the author and editor do not assume and hereby disclaim any liability to any party for any loss, damage, or disruption caused by errors or omissions, whether such errors or omissions result from negligence, accident, or any other cause.

This handbook is not intended as a substitute for the medical advice of physicians. The reader should regularly consult a physician in matters relating to his/her health and particularly with respect to any symptoms that may require diagnosis, medical attention, or behavioral therapy.

LIMITED DUPLICATION LICENSE

The author grants to individual purchasers of *Meal Planning Strategies, Tips, & Techniques - A Practical Handbook For Everyone,* nonassignable permission to reproduce these materials. This license is limited to you, the individual purchaser, for personal use or for use with clients in a professional setting. It does not extend to additional providers or practice settings, nor does purchase by an institution constitute a site license. This license does not grant the right to reproduce these materials for resale, redistribution, electronic display, or any other purposes (including but not limited to books, pamphlets, articles, video or audio tapes, blogs, file-sharing sites, internet or intranet sites, and handouts or slides for lectures, workshops, or webinars, whether or not a fee is charged). Permission to reproduce these materials for these and any other purposes must be obtained in writing from the author.

Kristine Sinner, MS, RDN, CEDRD
HowToMealPlan.com | KristineSinnerRDN.com

Edited and designed by Jessica Garvar, Wise Mind Marketing
WiseMindMarketing.com

First edition paperback & digital PDF, March 2019

ISBN: 978-1-7338404-0-8 (spiral bound)

This handbook is dedicated to all of my clients past, present, and future. You mean more to me than you will ever know.

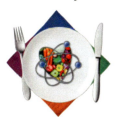

A Message From Kristine

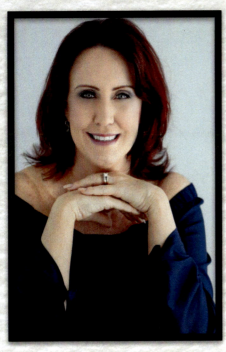

While the majority of my career has been spent treating eating disorder clients, it has always been a goal of mine to find a way to educate the masses. Whether or not a person has a clinical need to see me, year after year there has always been one thing that nearly every single one of them has said the second their toosh hits the couch in my office..."*Just Tell Me What To Eat!*" It is the phrase every dietitian in the world dreads to hear because what it really means is that the person more than likely believes they have little to no clue what they should eat. They usually believe that they know what they want to eat and then are overwhelmed by judgements of those wants based on everything other than the truth, the facts, or the science of nutrition.

As a society we have very little faith in our own food choices and everything is considered either good or bad. We were either never taught basic nutrition principles or after years of confusing messages from a $60 billion diet industry, not knowing which way is up has become far too normal. Expecting there is some secret all encompassing solution and coming to see the dietitian means they will finally be 'in the know' is also one of the biggest misconceptions. It follows suit with the idea that being a certain size or looking a certain way will make us happy. It's all maddening and what is both sad and relieving is that all along the answers we are desperate to find externally, actually lie within each and every one of us.

We are born knowing what we need and are taught to ignore it. Over time we lose the innate ability to connect to the notion that our bodies have all the answers. Intuitive hunger cues are totally foreign and eating is often a reactionary activity based off of having, needing, or yearning for an emotion of some sort. As a result we put more energy, focus, and years of our lives into the exploration of myths, fads, and misperceptions regarding nutrition because they appease to our need for urgency and emotional regulation. As a result, the irrefutable science of nutrition has been blown out the window and what blew in was desperation, deprivation, confusion, and quite often shame.

This handbook is 3 decades of helping clients to re-learn, and oftentimes learn for the very first time, the actual FACTS about Science Based Nutrition that have withstood the test of time, social trends, and generations of fad diets. As an <u>anti-diet dietitian</u> who strongly believes in reconnecting with our innate food and body connections that we are born knowing, my true hope is that this handbook will help end the voices in so many peoples' heads that confuse them, tear them down, cause them to treat lies as facts, and make food anything more than what is was ever intended to be...Fuel For Our Bodies!

This is a guide for EVERYONE and intended to be used with the whole family. This handbook is really everything you will ever need to know regarding your diet, so please let the insanity end here. I hereby officially release you of all the confusion you've acquired from years of dieting and believing endless false promises from each and every celebrity trend and food myth you've come across. Stop the diets and remove the word entirely from your vocabulary. Put your trust in me. Believe in my commitment to the field of dietetics, my passion to educate, and my desire to genuinely help change the conversation. My hope is that this handbook will affect you and give you the permission you need to reset your nutritional health.

Learn *#HowToMealPlan* and fuel your body to live the best life possible!

In Good Health,

Kristine J Sinner

Kristine Sinner, MS, RDN, CEDRD

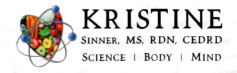

Use the hashtag *#HowToMealPlan* on social media to ask questions, post pictures, and share ideas!

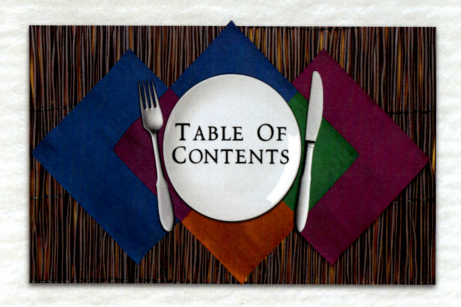

INTRODUCTION

PAGE		PAGE	
1	For REAL People Who Want To Be Healthy	2	Achieve A Healthier & Happier You
3	How to Use This Handbook	4	Meal Planning Approaches
5	8 Steps to Make the Best Use of This Handbook		

SECTION I: VARIETY, BALANCE, & MODERATION

PAGE		PAGE	
6	The Energy Yielding Nutrients	7	The Ideal Meal Setting
8	Food Choice Selections By Food Group	9	High Quality "Nutrient Rich" Food Sources
10	Nutrients Found in a Rainbow of Foods	11-15	Benefits of Eating a Rainbow of Foods
16	Best Food Choice From a Rainbow of Foods	17	A Well Balanced Meal Plan
18	The Ideal "Nutrient Rich" Well Balanced Meal Plan	19	Sample "Nutrient Rich" Well Balanced Meal Plan
20	Tips For Successful Meal Planning	21	Guidelines For Successful Meal Planning
22	What Counts As A Serving	23	Visualizing Portion Sizes
24	Portion Control Tips	25-28	Meal & Snack Ideas

SECTION II: SHOPPING & COOKING

PAGE		PAGE	
29	Nutrition at the Grocery Store	30	The 4 P's: Plan, Purchase, Prep, & Pack
31-4	Grocery Store "Best Picks"	35	Nutritious Pantry Basics
36	Nutritious Countertop Basics	37	Nutritious Refrigerator Basics
38	Nutritious Freezer Basics		

SECTION III: EATING AWAY FROM HOME

PAGE		PAGE	
39-41	Restaurant Eating Tips & Suggestions	42	Holidays, Vacations, and Special Occasions
43	What to Bring or Make on Holidays	44	Foods To Bring On Vacation

SECTION IV: PUTTING IT ALL TOGETHER

PAGE		PAGE	
45	How To Get Started	46	Planning For A Busy Week
47	The Dedicated Planning Hour	48	Shopping Day
49	Prepping Your Weekly Staples	50-51	Organizing Your Groceries For Optimal Usage
52	Refrigerator Single Serve Grab-n-Go Items	53	Pantry Single Serve Grab-n-Go Items

APPENDIX: MEAL PLANNING FORMS & INVENTORIES

PAGE		PAGE	
54-55	My Grocery List	56	Master Inventory List
57	What I PLAN TO EAT This Week	58	What I ATE This Week

INTRODUCTION

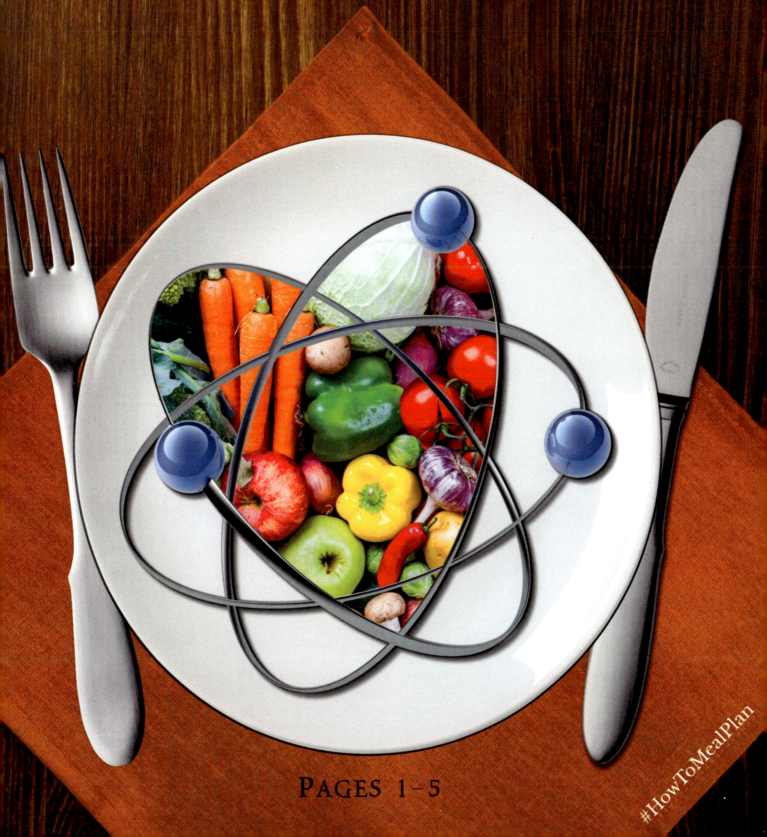

PAGES 1–5

INTRODUCTION

For REAL People Who WANT To LIVE Healthy

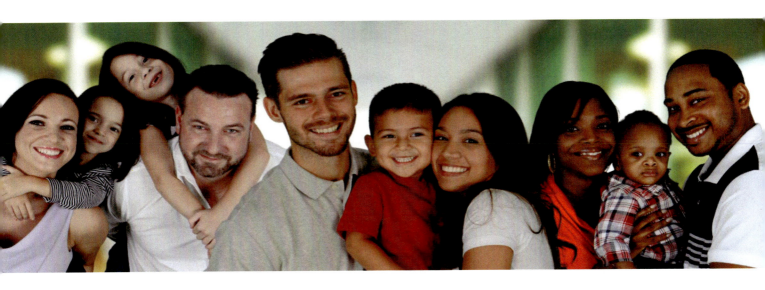

This meal planning handbook is a rare collection of all the educational handouts and strategies used for over 3 decades of nutrition counseling by an Expert Registered Dietitian and Medical Nutrition Therapist. On its own, it provides simple nutrition education as well as a resource for easy meal and snack ideas for the entire family. When used with a Registered Dietitian or other trained professional to individualize your nutrition, you will be armed with all of the most effective tools and resources needed to best maximize your time. Either way, you now have in your hands the irrefutable facts about all things nutrition that will serve as a foundation for achieving the healthy diet and ideal body weight for you and those you love.

Unlike many expensive diet programs, the goal of this handbook is to provide sound, science based nutrition education. All of the information shared is the simplification of proven research and applied practice theories that have stood the test of time. It is intended to help those who use it to move passed expensive and mentally exhausting diet trends and fads promoted by people without a scholarly education or applied practice experience to back their claims.

This handbook is not meant to be a substitute for nutrition counseling by a Registered Dietitian and is not designed to address specific disease states, as those can only be diagnosed by a medical professional. If you would like information that is more tailored to your individual needs, you are welcomed to schedule a virtual consult with Kristine Sinner, MS, RDN at:

HowToMealPlan.com

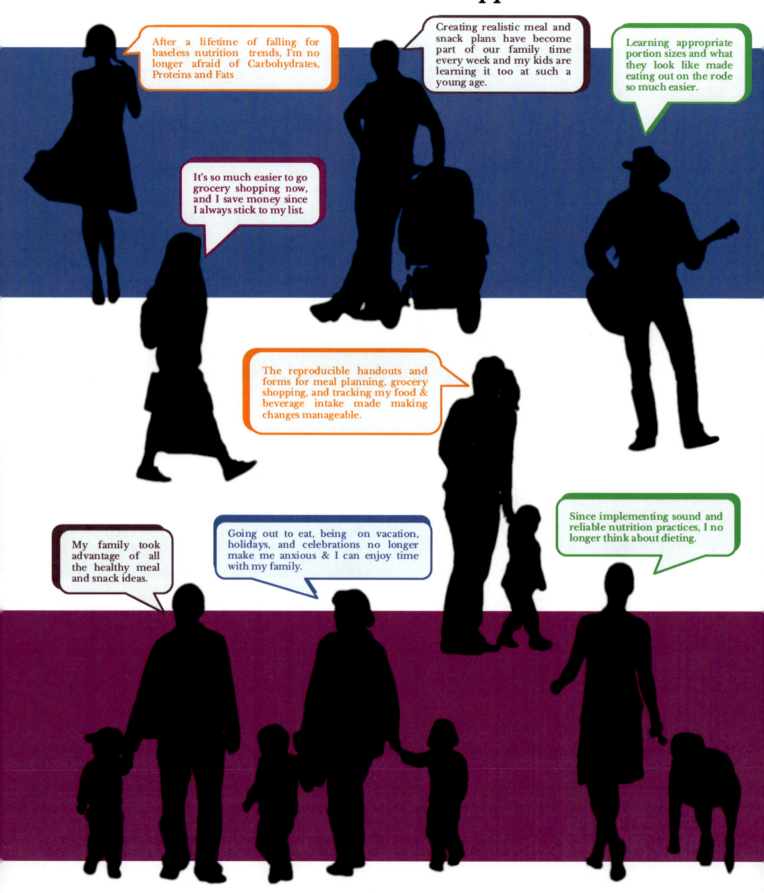

INTRODUCTION

#HowToMealPlan

How To Use This Handbook:

In the appendix of this handbook you will find several forms and lists to help you throughout the meal planning process. You are welcomed to make copies for personal usage as often as you like. When used consistently, these forms and lists will prove to be a tremendous help to you and your family as you manage the day to day needs that arise in order to maintain and/or achieve your nutritional goals. Absorb yourself into the following pages and you will find all of the best and most reliable tools and information needed to develop a nutritionally complete and functional meal and snack plan to use as a foundation for lifelong healthy eating habits.

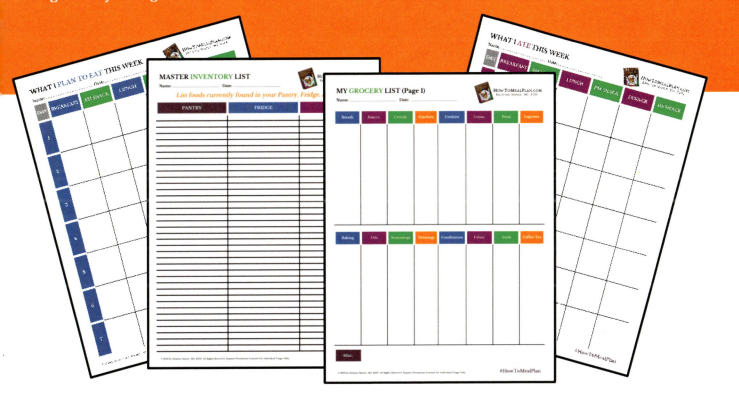

First, a basic meal plan framework will be provided which can be applied to every member of your family at any age. Next, you will be given tips on:

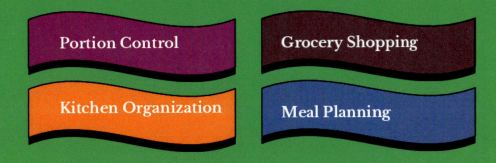

- Portion Control
- Grocery Shopping
- Kitchen Organization
- Meal Planning

MEAL PLANNING STRATEGIES, TIPS, & TECHNIQUES | WRITTEN BY: KRISTINE SINNER, MS, RDN

INTRODUCTION

#HowToMealPlan

Meal Planning Approaches

This handbook provides basic nutrition information as well as a variety of different tools that can be used to plan meals. If you are working with a dietitian or other trained professional they will help you choose a meal plan approach that is best suited to your particular needs. If you are using this handbook on your own as a useful reference tool, you can elect to choose one of the following meal planning strategies to best suit your needs. Once you choose your meal planning approach, less structured or more structured, you can then use the rest of the manual to guide you through the process of incorporating the changes needed to achieve a healthier lifestyle for you and your family.

Less Structured

The Simple Plate Meal Plan Method (Page 6):

This method utilizes a visual tool of the salad plate (Approx. 6-8") to typify the "ideal meal setup". The plate is divided into three sections. ½ of the plate is to be filled with vegetables, ¼ of the plate is to include a lean protein source, and the remaining ¼ of the plate is to include a grain or other carbohydrate source. An added fat serving may be included on the plate as you desire. This meal is rounded off with the inclusion of a serving of dairy and fruit to provide a complete and nutrient rich meal. It is recommended that a snack be added each day between meals that contains either a lean protein or dairy source, coupled with a complex carbohydrate or fruit source.

More Structured

The Six Small Meals Method (Pages 17-19):

You simply strive to get one food from each food group at meals and two to three food groups at snack. Snacks should have a least one protein containing food. There are more complex meal plan forms in Appendix A that you can use to either help you to track the number of foods you are eating from each food group, or that help you break down a specific pattern of the number of servings of each food group you would like to achieve at each meal . If you desire an individualized meal plan prescription, consider scheduling a consultation for a 1:1 session with a Registered Dietitian.

MEAL PLANNING STRATEGIES, TIPS, & TECHNIQUES | WRITTEN BY: KRISTINE SINNER, MS, RDN

INTRODUCTION

#HowToMealPlan

8 Steps to Make the Best Use of This Handbook

1. Read Section I & II

2. Get familiarized with portion sizes and the 4P's, a key strategy for meal planning success.

3. Choose your preferred approach for your meal planning. (page 4)

4. Review and consider which nutrients you may be lacking and then include them into your meal plan.

5. Read through all of the meal and snack ideas as well as the grocery store best picks and tips.

6. Use the forms in the appendix to create your grocery list and plan a week of meals and snacks.

7. Bring this handbook with you when you go grocery shopping in case any questions arise.

8. Portion, prep, and pack your groceries as needed for you and your family. ENJOY!

MEAL PLANNING STRATEGIES, TIPS, & TECHNIQUES | WRITTEN BY: KRISTINE SINNER, MS, RDN

SECTION 1
Variety, Balance, & Moderation

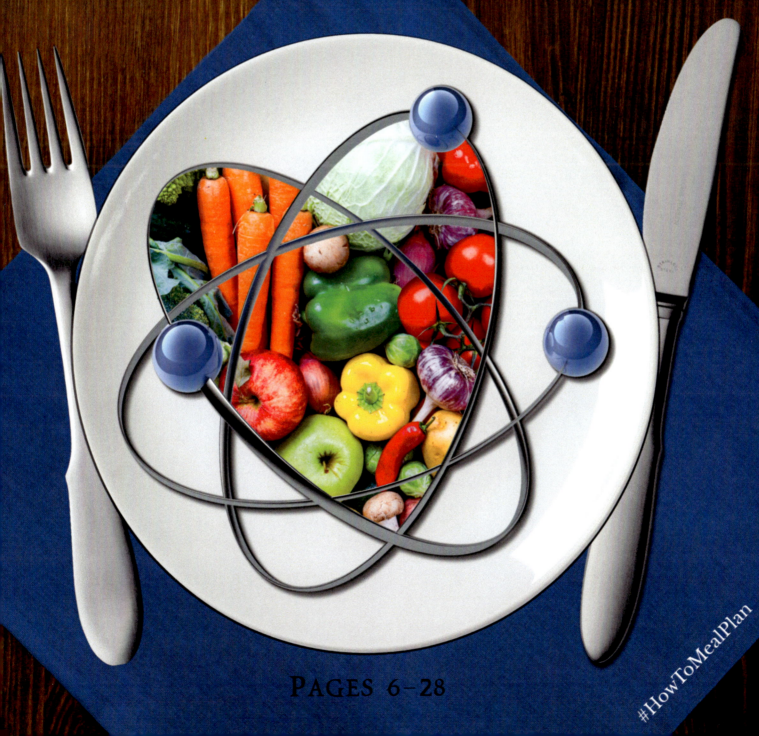

PAGES 6–28

#HowToMealPlan

VARIETY, BALANCE, & MODERATION

#HowToMealPlan

The Energy Yielding Nutrients

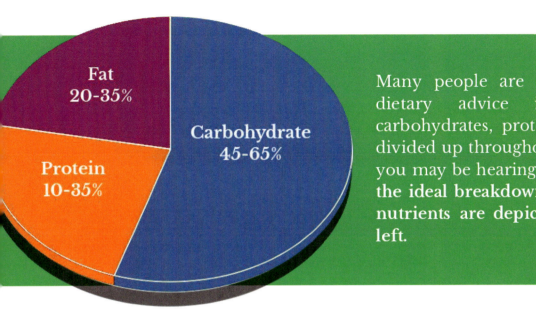

Many people are confused by conflicting dietary advice in regards to how carbohydrates, proteins, and fats should be divided up throughout the day. Despite what you may be hearing from the latest fad diets, the ideal breakdown of the energy yielding nutrients are depicted by the chart to the left.

CARBOHYDRATE:

The PRIMARY source of energy for the body! Carbohydrate is the first food fuel source used and metabolized by the body for mechanical and mental energy. Its energy is provided to us in our diet through starches/breads, dairy, fruits and vegetables. As a result, approximately 45 to 65 % of our total daily calorie intake should come from this energy filled nutrient. Our bodies absolutely depend on carbohydrates to provide us with adequate energy and to allow for maintenance of a consistent and stable bodyweight.

PROTEIN:

The body uses Protein to build and maintain lean muscle, the integrity of vital organs. and to maintain vital protein pools. It is also used to make other critical body substances that control body functions. For a majority of meal plans, Protein will provide 10-35% of your daily caloric intake. More is not better. It is not necessary to overdo this macronutrient as the body will only use what it needs and excrete the rest. Any caloric excess regardless of the source will be seen by the body as unnecessary and can be stored as fat.

FAT:

This macronutrient is the SECOND most preferred source of energy for the body. Fat in the diet is absolutely essential for proper body functioning. Fats are needed to maintain healthy skin, hair, and eyes. They are also used to make hormones that are critical for proper brain function and memory as well as to carry fat-soluble vitamins. About 20 to 35% of meal plan calories ARE REQUIRED from this nutrient to maintain optimal daily health. Providing our bodies with adequate amounts of carbohydrate and fat makes it possible for the body to spare protein for other uses such as muscle building, maintenance, and repair versus being used as an energy source.

---

*Source- U.S. Department of Health and Human Services and U.S. Department of Agriculture. 2015 – 2020 Dietary Guidelines for Americans. 8th Edition. December 2015. Available at https://health.gov/dietaryguidelines/2015/guidelines

VARIETY, BALANCE, & MODERATION

#HowToMealPlan

The Ideal Meal Setting (6-8" Plate)

Fruit
Choose a variety of bright, deeply colored fruits as much as possible. Explore new textures and uses like cubed, sliced, strips, & dried. Fresh (with skin on) when possible & buy frozen for nutrient packed smoothies. Pre-cut fruit trays are a great options for a simple and convenient way to cut down on prep time when needed.

Dairy
Milk, dairy free alternatives, kefir, cheese, cottage cheese (try single serve 4-packs for convenience), ricotta cheese, ice cream, and yogurt

Added Fats
Margarine, butter, avocado, olives, or hummus. Try extra virgin and cold pressed oils (olive, canola, avocado, sunflower, walnut, flaxseed). All raw nuts, seeds, hemp chia seeds and flax

Grains/Starches
100% whole grain, wheat, oat, rye, barley, farro, millet, rice, quinoa, or bulgur. Have a goal for 3-4g fiber/serving or 25-38 total grams fiber/day.

Vegetables
Choose fresh produce when possible and prepare fresh, steamed, roasted, or grilled. Keep a variety of bright, deep colors and textures. Leave the skin on when possible, and when needed purchase pre-cut trays for added convenience.

Protein
Lean beef, chicken, turkey, fish, game, or bison. Try legumes, beans and peas as well as fatty fish 2-3 times/week. Whole nuts and nut butters, meatless alternatives, eggs, and any other egg substitutes.

Meal Planning Strategies, Tips, & Techniques | Written By: Kristine Sinner, MS, RDN

VARIETY, BALANCE, & MODERATION #HowToMealPlan

Food Choice Selections By Food Group

Dairy
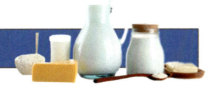

Regular Milk
All Types of Cheese- *Block, Cubed, String, Shredded, Spreads*
Dairy-Free Milk Alternatives- *Soy, Almond, Cashew, Oat, Coconut*

Yogurt
Greek Yogurt
Kefir
Cottage Cheese
Ricotta Cheese

Grains

Whole Grain (≥3-4g *fiber/svg*): *Bread, Rice, Pasta, Crackers, Rolls, Cereals, Tortillas*
Legumes: *Lentils, Various Whole Beans (Black, Pinto, Garbanzo, Cannellini, Kidney, Edamame*

Whole Grain Muffins
Whole Grain Pancakes
Whole Grain Waffles
Potatoes

Protein
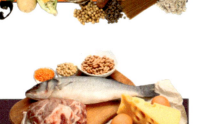

Very Lean, Lean, or Low-Fat Meats- *Chicken, Turkey, Fish, Game, Bison*
Vegetarian/Meat Alternatives
Deli Meats and Cheeses
Eggs/Egg Substitute
Legumes/Beans- *Peas, Edamame, Garbanzo, Black, Kidney, Lentils*

Natural Nut/Seed Spreads- *Peanut, Cashew, Almond, Sunflower*
Shellfish/Fish Fillet- *Wild Caught Salmon, Cod, Sea Bass, Mahi Mahi, Halibut, Trout*
Cottage Cheese, Ricotta cheese
Hummus
Protein & Peanut Butter Powder
Tofu

Fruits & Vegetables
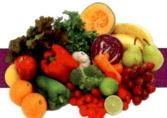

Ideally Any Whole, Fresh, Frozen, or Canned in Water Fruits & Vegetables

Any Fresh Juices With Pulp
Unsweetened Dried Fruit

Fat

Olives
Nuts & Seeds
Oils- *Olive, Canola, Sunflower, Sesame, Flax*
Unsalted Butter or Trans Fat Free Margarine
Canola or Olive Oil Based Salad Dressings

Natural Peanut Butter
Hemp+
Shredded Coconut
Avocado
Flaxseeds

Fun/Recreational
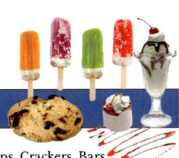

Think Kids or Lunch-Box Size
Prepackaged or Pre-portioned Cookies, Cakes, Pies, Muffins, Pudding, Ice Cream
Single-serve, Individually Portioned Candies

Lunch Box Bag Sized Snack Chips, Crackers, Bars, Nuts
Small Size Specialty Coffees, Lattes, Frozen Blended Drinks

MEAL PLANNING STRATEGIES, TIPS, & TECHNIQUES | WRITTEN BY: KRISTINE SINNER, MS, RDN

VARIETY, BALANCE, & MODERATION
#HowToMealPlan

High Quality "Nutrient Rich" Food Sources

Soluble Fiber

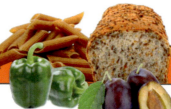

Oat Bran
Oatmeal
Lentils and Peas
Beans (Black and Kidney)
Cabbage

Brussels Sprouts
Citrus Fruit, Pears, Plums
Apple, Blackberries, Raisins
Broccoli
Carrots

Insoluble Fiber

Whole Wheat, Barley, Quinoa, Farro
Whole Multigrain Breads, Rolls and Pitas
Ground Psyllium Seeds
Whole Grain Pasta
Black, Brown, & Red Rice
Legumes

Rolled Oats
Wheat Bran
Rice Bran
Wheat Germ
Raw Fruit
Fruits and Vegetables with Skin

Healthy Fats

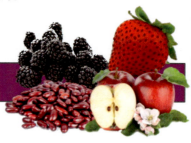

Oils - *Olive, Canola, Peanut, Sesame, Walnut, Soybean, Flaxseed, Grape Seed*
Nuts - *Macadamia, Hazelnuts, Pecans, Almonds, Cashews, Pistachios, Brazil, Peanuts, Pine, Walnuts*
Seeds- *Sesame, Chia, Sunflower, Hemp*

Spreads - *Peanut Butter, Almond Butter, Cashew Butter, Tahini/Sesame Butter, Sunflower Seed Butter*
Black and Green Olives
Avocado
Dark Chocolate

Antioxidants

Wild Blueberries, Goji Berries, Acai, Blackberries, Raspberries
Red Kidney and Pinto Beans
Cranberries, Pomegranate, Grapes
Artichokes, Kale, Red Cabbage

Dried Prunes
Strawberries
Red Apples
Wild Cherries
Dark Chocolate

Omega 3 Fatty Acids | Long-Chain Fatty Acids | Omega 6 Fatty Acids

Oils- *Krill, Canola, Flax, Hemp, Algal, & Walnut*
Seeds- *Hemp, Chia, Sesame & Flax*
Black Walnuts
Edamame

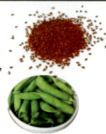

Salmon
Mackerel
Tuna
Herring
Sardines
Fortified Eggs, Yogurt, Kefir & Milk

Soybean Oil
Sunflower Oil
Sunflower Seeds
Corn Oil
Canola Margarines
Salad Dressing
Olive Oil Mayo

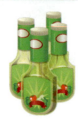

*Source- U.S. Department of Health and Human Services and U.S. Department of Agriculture. 2015 – 2020 Dietary Guidelines for Americans. 8th Edition. December 2015. Available at https://health.gov/dietaryguidelines/2015/guidelines

---

MEAL PLANNING STRATEGIES, TIPS, & TECHNIQUES | WRITTEN BY: KRISTINE SINNER, MS, RDN

VARIETY, BALANCE, & MODERATION
#HowToMealPlan

Nutrients Found In A *RAINBOW* of Foods

There Is More To Consider Than Just Calories!

DETOXIFICATION	IMMUNE SUPPORT	CANCER PREVENTION	HEART HEALTH	LONGEVITY
Flavones	Beta-Glucans	Beta-cryptoxanthin	Anthocyanidins	Lutein
Flavanones	EGCG SDG	Flavonols	Flavonols	Zeaxanthin
Flavanols	Lignans	Flavanones	Flavones	Resveratrol Vit. C
Zeaxanthin	Indoles	Alpha-Carotene	Flavan-3-ols	Fiber Flavonoids
Indoles	Isothiocyanates	Beta-Carotene	Proanthocyanidins	Flavan-3-ols
Isothiocyanates	Organosulfur Compounds	Zeaxanthin	Lycopene	Ellagic Acid Quercetin
Fiber		Lycopene	Ellagic Acid Quercetin Hesperidin	Proanthocyanidins
Lutein		Potassium Vitamin C	Resveratrol	
Zeaxanthin				
Organosulfur Compounds				
Beta-Carotene				

Source: Phytochemical Info Center, Phytochemical List- https://pbhfoundation.org/about/res/pic/phytolist#

MEAL PLANNING STRATEGIES, TIPS, & TECHNIQUES | WRITTEN BY: KRISTINE SINNER, MS, RDN

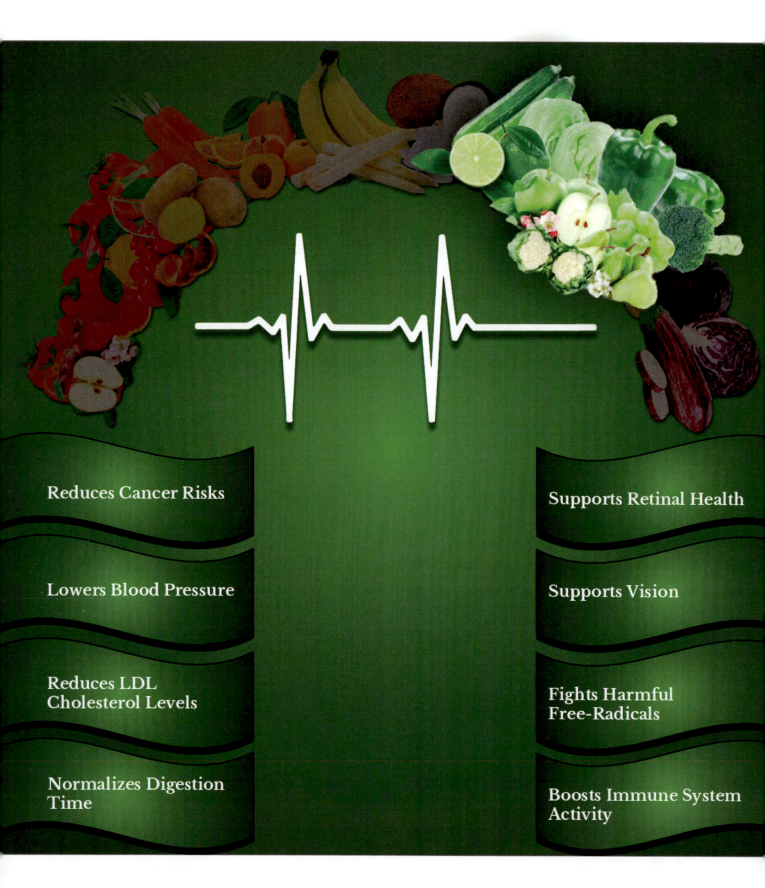

VARIETY, BALANCE, & MODERATION
#HowToMealPlan

Benefits of Eating WHITE Fruits & Vegetables

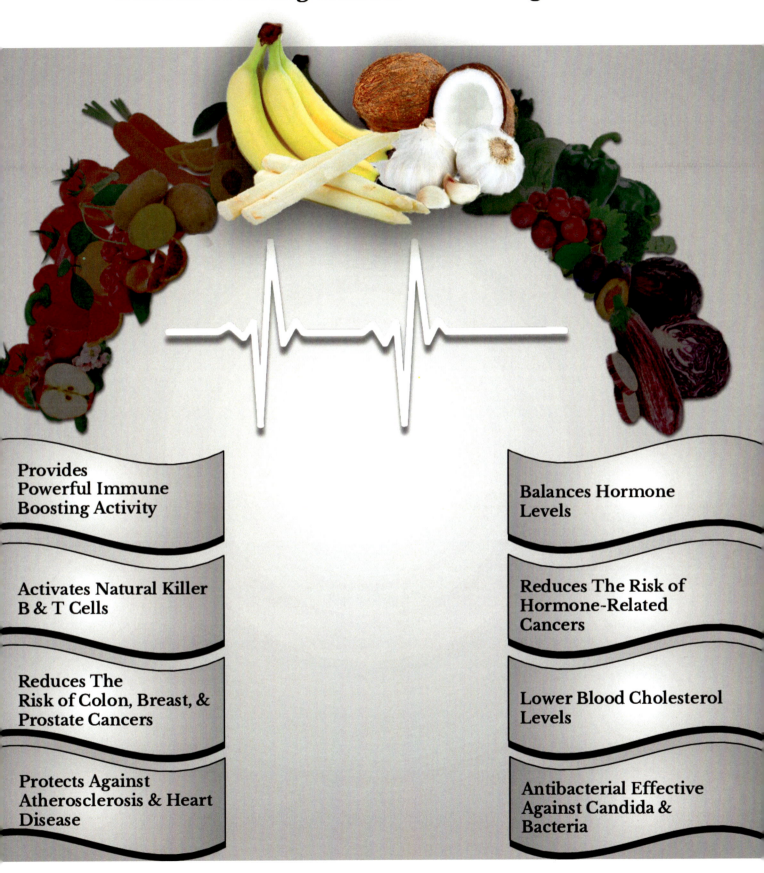

- Provides Powerful Immune Boosting Activity
- Activates Natural Killer B & T Cells
- Reduces The Risk of Colon, Breast, & Prostate Cancers
- Protects Against Atherosclerosis & Heart Disease

- Balances Hormone Levels
- Reduces The Risk of Hormone-Related Cancers
- Lower Blood Cholesterol Levels
- Antibacterial Effective Against Candida & Bacteria

*Source: Phytochemical Info Center, Phytochemical List- https://pbhfoundation.org/about/res/pic/phytolist#

MEAL PLANNING STRATEGIES, TIPS, & TECHNIQUES | WRITTEN BY: KRISTINE SINNER, MS, RDN

VARIETY, BALANCE, & MODERATION
#HowToMealPlan

Benefits of Eating RED Fruits & Vegetables

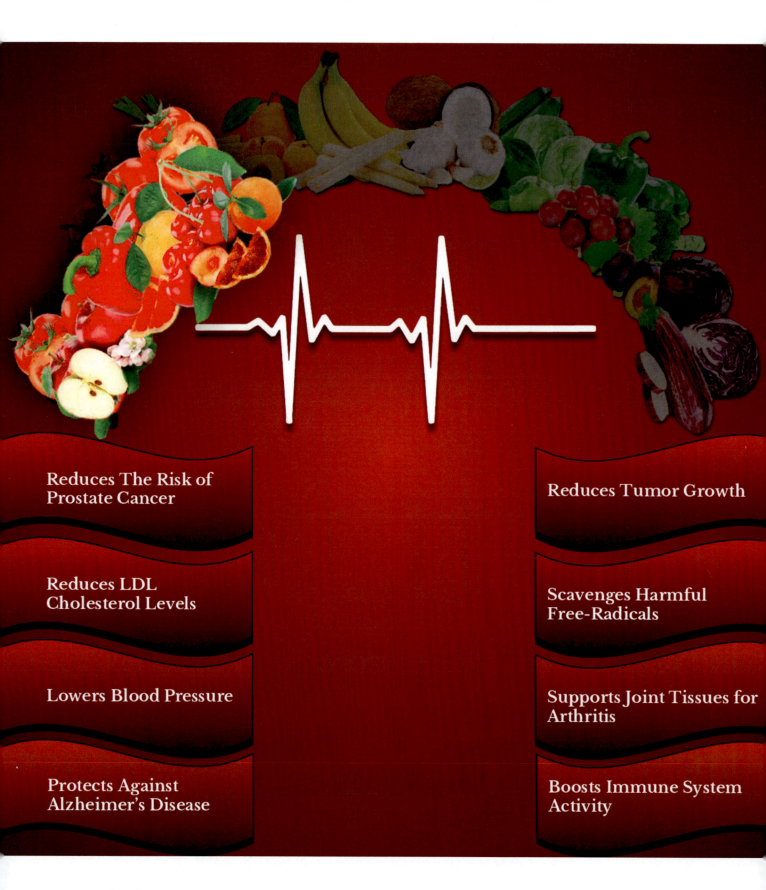

- Reduces The Risk of Prostate Cancer
- Reduces LDL Cholesterol Levels
- Lowers Blood Pressure
- Protects Against Alzheimer's Disease

- Reduces Tumor Growth
- Scavenges Harmful Free-Radicals
- Supports Joint Tissues for Arthritis
- Boosts Immune System Activity

*Source: Phytochemical Info Center, Phytochemical List- https://pbhfoundation.org/about/res/pic/phytolist#

MEAL PLANNING STRATEGIES, TIPS, & TECHNIQUES | WRITTEN BY: KRISTINE SINNER, MS, RDN

VARIETY, BALANCE, & MODERATION
#HowToMealPlan

Benefits of Eating YELLOW/ORANGE Fruits & Vegetables

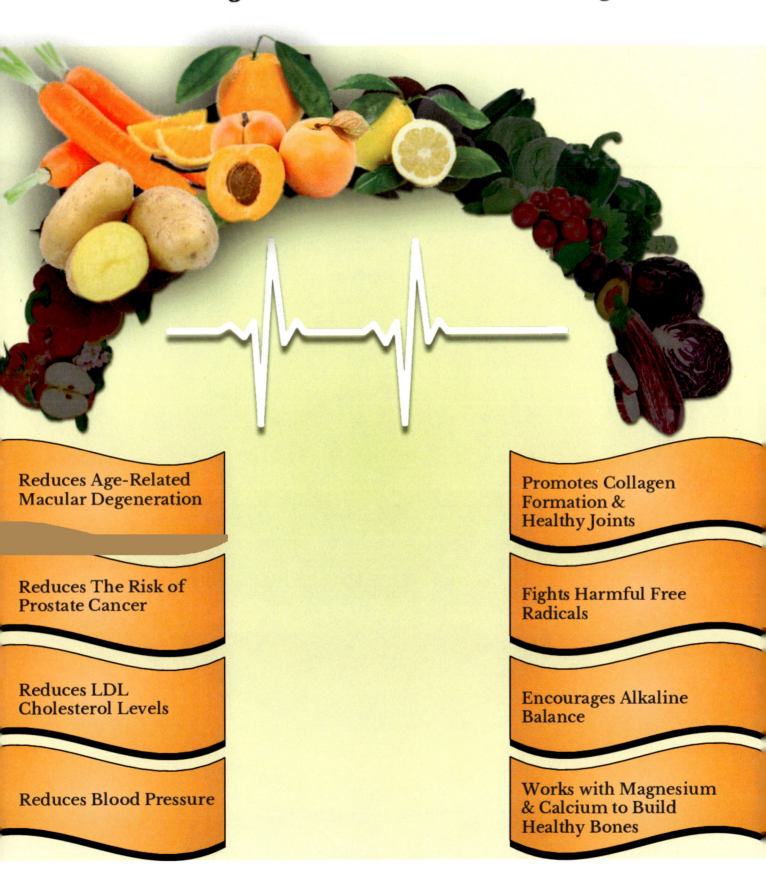

- Reduces Age-Related Macular Degeneration
- Reduces The Risk of Prostate Cancer
- Reduces LDL Cholesterol Levels
- Reduces Blood Pressure

- Promotes Collagen Formation & Healthy Joints
- Fights Harmful Free Radicals
- Encourages Alkaline Balance
- Works with Magnesium & Calcium to Build Healthy Bones

*Source: Phytochemical Info Center, Phytochemical List- https://pbhfoundation.org/about/res/pic/phytolist#

MEAL PLANNING STRATEGIES, TIPS, & TECHNIQUES | WRITTEN BY: KRISTINE SINNER, MS, RDN

VARIETY, BALANCE, & MODERATION
#HowToMealPlan

Benefits of Eating BLUE/PURPLE Fruits & Vegetables

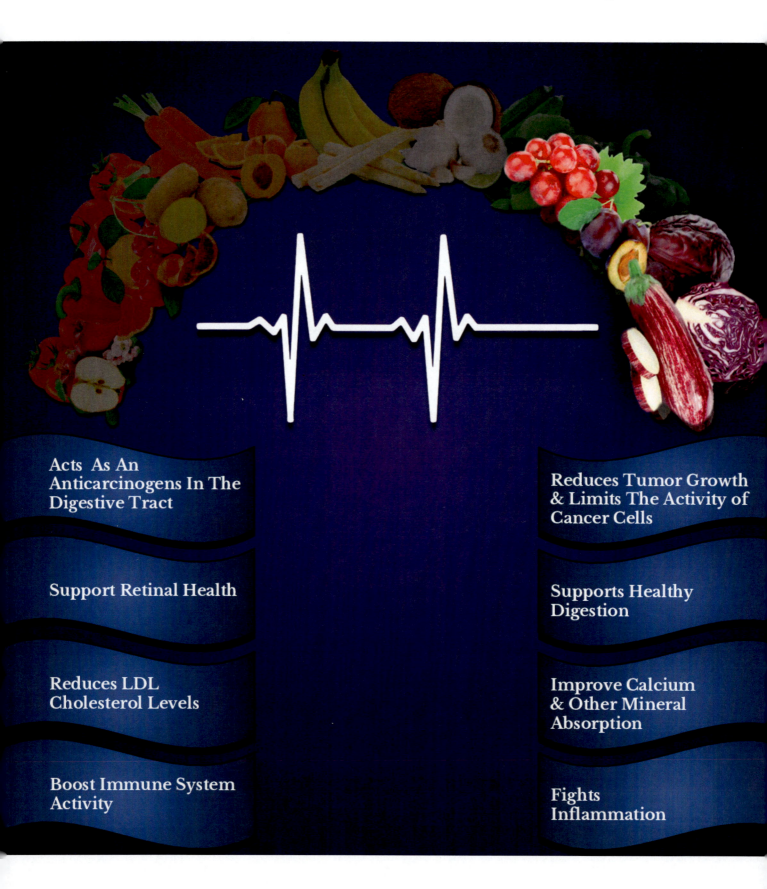

- Acts As An Anticarcinogens In The Digestive Tract
- Support Retinal Health
- Reduces LDL Cholesterol Levels
- Boost Immune System Activity

- Reduces Tumor Growth & Limits The Activity of Cancer Cells
- Supports Healthy Digestion
- Improve Calcium & Other Mineral Absorption
- Fights Inflammation

*Source: Phytochemical Info Center, Phytochemical List- https://pbhfoundation.org/about/res/pic/phytolist#

MEAL PLANNING STRATEGIES, TIPS, & TECHNIQUES | WRITTEN BY: KRISTINE SINNER, MS, RDN

VARIETY, BALANCE, & MODERATION
#HowToMealPlan

Best Food Choices From A RAINBOW of Foods

Green

- Artichokes
- Arugula
- Asparagus
- Avocados
- Broccoflower
- Broccoli
- Broccoli Rabe
- Brussel Sprouts
- Celery
- Chayote Squash
- Chinese Cabbage
- Cucumbers
- Endive
- Green Apples
- Green Beans
- Green Cabbage
- Green Grapes
- Green Onion
- Green Pears
- Green Peppers
- Honeydew
- Kiwifruit
- Leafy Greens
- Leeks
- Lettuce
- Limes
- Okra
- Peas
- Snow Peas
- Spinach
- Sugar Snap Peas
- Watercress
- Zucchini

White

- Bananas
- Brown Pears
- Cauliflower
- Dates
- Garlic
- Ginger
- Jerusalem Artichoke
- Jicama
- Kohlrabi
- Mushrooms
- Onions
- Parsnips
- Potatoes
- Shallots
- Turnips
- White Corn
- White Nectarines
- White peaches

Yellow/Orange

- Apricots
- Butternut Squash
- Cantaloupe
- Cape Gooseberries
- Carrots
- Golden Kiwifruit
- Grapefruit
- Lemon
- Mangoes
- Nectarines
- Oranges
- Papayas
- Peaches
- Persimmons
- Pineapples
- Pumpkin
- Rutabagas
- Sweet Corn
- Sweet Potatoes
- Tangerines
- Yellow Apples
- Yellow Beets
- Yellow Figs
- Yellow Winter Squash
- Yellow Pear
- Yellow Peppers
- Yellow Potatoes
- Yellow Summer Squash
- Yellow Tomatoes
- Yellow Watermelon

Red

- Beets
- Blood Oranges
- Cherries
- Cranberries
- Guava
- Papaya
- Pink Grapefruit
- Pink/Red Grapefruit
- Pomegranates
- Radicchio
- Radishes
- Raspberries
- Red Apples
- Red Bell Peppers
- Red Chili Peppers
- Red Grapes
- Red Onions
- Red Pears
- Red Peppers
- Red Potatoes
- Rhubarb
- Strawberries
- Tomatoes
- Watermelon

Blue/Purple

- Raisins
- Prunes
- Purple Peppers
- Elderberries
- Black Currants
- Red Onions
- Cherries
- Purple Artichokes
- Purple Kale
- Purple Belgian Endive
- Radicchio
- Purple Broccoli
- Purple Basil
- Pluots
- Edible Violets
- Red Leaf Lettuce
- Purple Thyme
- Purple Kohlrabi
- Microgreens

*Source- USDA National Nutrient Database For Standard Reference Legacy Release, April 2018

MEAL PLANNING STRATEGIES, TIPS, & TECHNIQUES | WRITTEN BY: KRISTINE SINNER, MS, RDN

VARIETY, BALANCE, & MODERATION

#HowToMealPlan

A Well Balanced Meal Plan

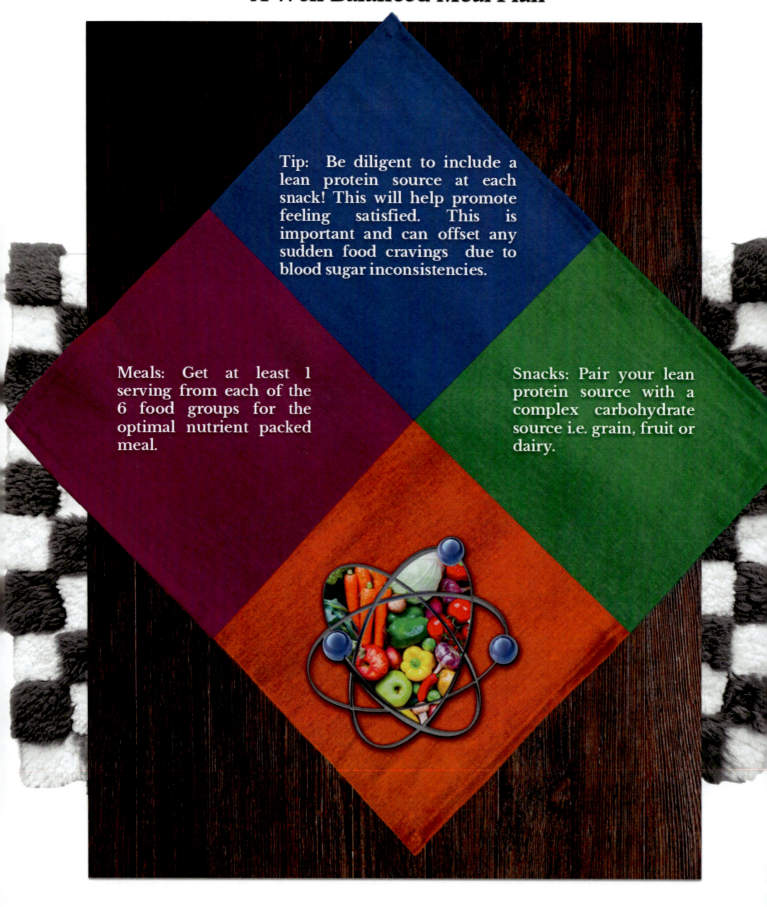

Tip: Be diligent to include a lean protein source at each snack! This will help promote feeling satisfied. This is important and can offset any sudden food cravings due to blood sugar inconsistencies.

Meals: Get at least 1 serving from each of the 6 food groups for the optimal nutrient packed meal.

Snacks: Pair your lean protein source with a complex carbohydrate source i.e. grain, fruit or dairy.

MEAL PLANNING STRATEGIES, TIPS, & TECHNIQUES | WRITTEN BY: KRISTINE SINNER, MS, RDN

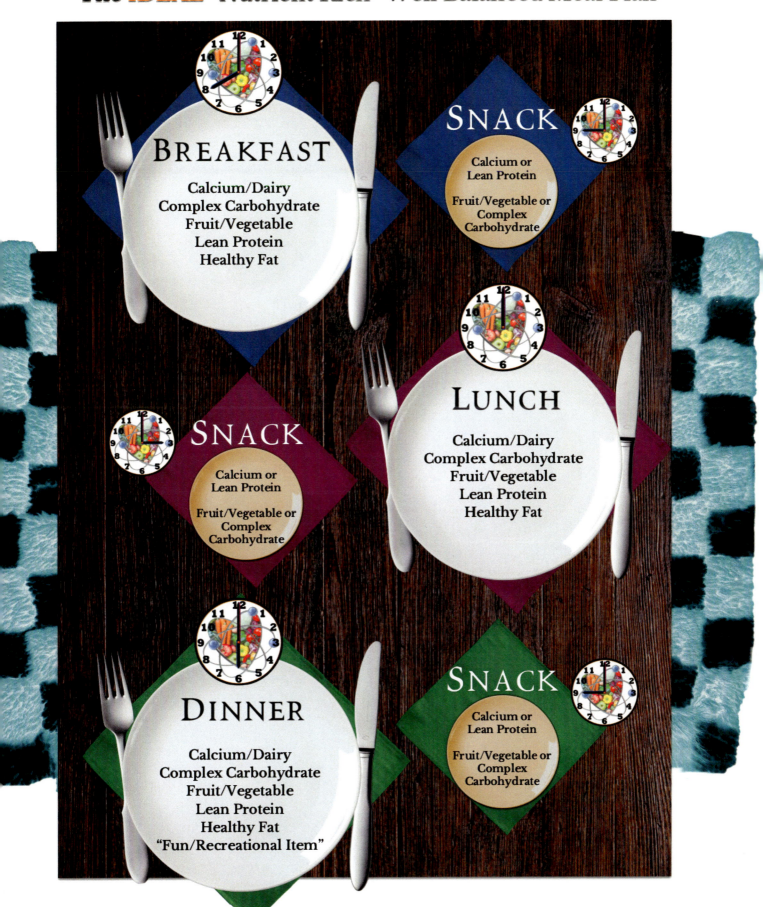

VARIETY, BALANCE, & MODERATION
#HowToMealPlan

SAMPLE "Nutrient-Rich" Well Balanced Meal Plan

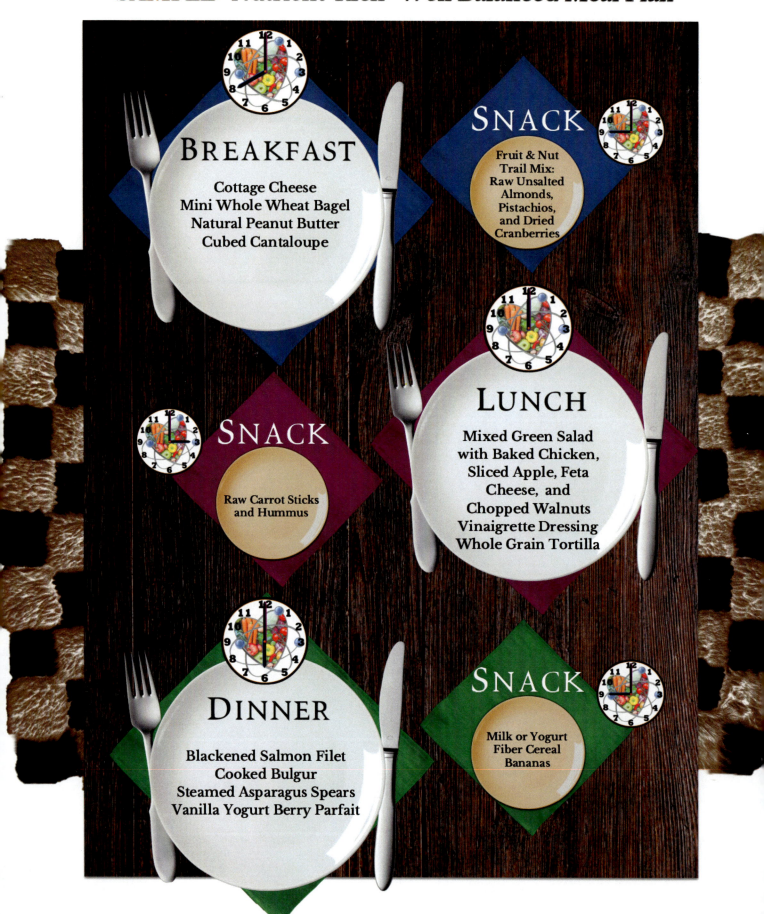

BREAKFAST
Cottage Cheese
Mini Whole Wheat Bagel
Natural Peanut Butter
Cubed Cantaloupe

SNACK
Fruit & Nut Trail Mix: Raw Unsalted Almonds, Pistachios, and Dried Cranberries

SNACK
Raw Carrot Sticks and Hummus

LUNCH
Mixed Green Salad with Baked Chicken, Sliced Apple, Feta Cheese, and Chopped Walnuts
Vinaigrette Dressing
Whole Grain Tortilla

DINNER
Blackened Salmon Filet
Cooked Bulgur
Steamed Asparagus Spears
Vanilla Yogurt Berry Parfait

SNACK
Milk or Yogurt
Fiber Cereal
Bananas

Meal Planning Strategies, Tips, & Techniques | Written By: Kristine Sinner, MS, RDN

VARIETY, BALANCE, & MODERATION

#HowToMealPlan

Tips For Successful Meal Planning

A successful meal plan is PRE-PLANNED to increase STRUCTURE and ORGANIZATION, as well as to decrease anxiety over what to eat. Follow these helpful tips when getting started.

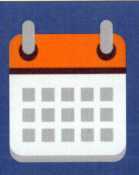
Pick a day of the week to plan a full week of meals and snacks, paying close attention to each day's schedule and plan accordingly.

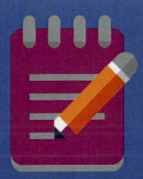
Complete a grocery list that coincides with your plan and includes all of the ingredients needed to make the recipes you selected for the week.

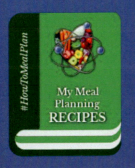
Look through your cookbooks, as well as online resources, for 3-4 recipes to prepare for the week.

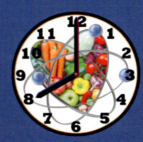
Plan for 3 meals and 2 to 3 snacks per day in order to avoid going longer than 3 to 4 hours without nourishment.

THESE TIPS WILL HELP TO ENSURE YOU ARE BEST EQUIPPED TO:

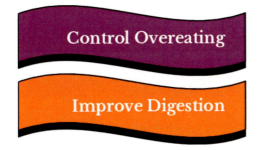

- Control Overeating
- Diversify Nutrition
- Improve Digestion
- Sustain Energy

Meal Planning Strategies, Tips, & Techniques | Written By: Kristine Sinner, MS, RDN

VARIETY, BALANCE, & MODERATION

#HowToMealPlan

Guidelines For Successful Meal Planning

SUCCESSFUL MEAL PLANS INCLUDE:

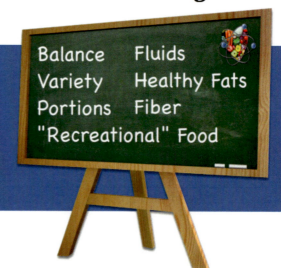

Balance   Fluids
Variety   Healthy Fats
Portions Fiber
"Recreational" Food

A balance from each of the six food groups. Ideally, each meal will include at least **(1) serving** from each group. All snacks will have at least one **complex carbohydrate** and one **lean protein** source. Including protein at every meal and snack helps to stabilize blood sugar, helps muscles to recover after exercise, and will offset food cravings later on.

A variety of foods within each of the six food groups. Alternate food choices within each food group to avoid monotony and ensure colorful, thus optimal nutrition. Choose a variety of colors and textures. Avoid repeating the same **meals or snacks** for three consecutive days when making meal plans. It is reasonable to repeat meals and snacks when on a budget and is common practice. The key is to rotate foods in and out often.

Approximate portion sizes. This will provide structure and consistency to the amount eaten, and will not promote the rigidity that can comes along with weighing and measuring. Flexibility allows for more or less of the foods you want vs. limiting yourself to strict amounts which can leave you feeling trapped and deprived, which increases the likelihood of overeating later on.

A suitable amount of fiber. Choose 100% whole grain breads, rice, ancient grains, and cereals whenever possible. Fiber is important for promoting satiety, bowel regularity, and optimal blood cholesterol levels.

A sufficient amount of monounsaturated fats, especially omega 3 rich fats and oils. A sufficient intake of fats are essential for the promotion of satiety, feeling of satisfaction, and optimal heart health Fat has the important role of carrying the flavor and enhancing the mouthfeel of food.

Adequate fluids to promote proper hydration, digestion, elimination of waste, and normal fluid balance. Everyone needs at least 8-15 cups of non-caffeinated fluids each day.

Some type of "recreational food" on a regular basis. Include the treats you like such as specialty coffees, sweets, chips, etc... This will prevent deprivation and the potential for bingeing.

Appropriate calories ensuring caloric levels NEVER go below 1,200 calories per day. For example, a normal caloric intake for an average woman is approximately 1500 to 1800 calories per day. Eating a very low calorie diet can promote an initial decrease in weight and is realistically not sustainable in the long run due to a resulting decrease in metabolic rate and or returning to eating the way you "used" to.

MEAL PLANNING STRATEGIES, TIPS, & TECHNIQUES | WRITTEN BY: KRISTINE SINNER, MS, RDN

VARIETY, BALANCE, & MODERATION #HowToMealPlan

What Counts As A Serving?

Dairy

1 cup Skim or 1% Milk
1 cup Yogurt Light or Plain
1 cup Greek Yogurt
¾ cup Cottage Cheese
2 teaspoon Grated Parmesan Cheese
1 oz. Cheese
1 oz. Ricotta Cheese
1 each String Cheese

Grains

1 Slice Whole Grain Bread
⅓ cup Cooked Brown Rice
1 Small Roll, Biscuit, Muffin
¾ cup Cold Breakfast Cereal
6 Small Crackers
3 Tbsps Wheat Germ
½ cup Cooked Cereal
6" Tortilla
½ cup Cooked Bulgur
⅓ cup Cooked Legumes
¾ oz. Pretzels
½ cup Bran Cereal
3 cup Air Popped Popcorn
3 oz. Baked White or Sweet Potato
⅓ cup Cooked Barley or Couscous
½ cup Green Peas, Corn or Sweet Potato
2 Slices Low Calorie/Lite Bread or Bagel Thins
½ Medium Bagel, Pita, Bun, English Muffin

Protein

1 oz. Skinless Poultry, Beef, or Fish
2 oz. Shellfish
2 oz. Canned Tuna in Water
1 cup Legumes, Cooked or Canned
1 scoop Protein Powder (15g/scoop)
1 oz. Cheese
2 Large Egg Whites
1 Whole Egg
2 Tbsp Peanut Butter (1 fat and 1 protein)
4 oz. Tofu

Fruits & Vegetables

1 Medium Apple, Orange, Kiwi
½ Banana, Mango, Grapefruit
¼ Wedge Melon 8"/ 1 cup Cubed Melon
1 cup Berries
½ cup Unsweetened Fruit Juice
½ cup Veg Juice
½ cup Grapes
½ cup Sliced Fruit or ¼ cup Dried Fruit
½ cup Cooked Vegetables
1 cup Raw Vegetables
2 Tbsps Raisins or Dried Cranberries

Fat

1 Tsp Liquid Oils or Tsp Butter or Margarine
2 Tsp Light Margarine
1 Tbsp Peanut Butter,
1 Tbsp Reduced Fat Mayo or Salad Dressing
1 Tbsp Cream Cheese or Sour Cream
2 Tbsp Lite Cream Cheese
1 ½ Tbsp Ground Flax Meal
⅛ of an Avocado
8 Lg Black Olives or 10 Green Stuffed Olives
½ cup Shelled Nuts

*Source: The Exchange Lists for Meal Planning, The American Diabetes Association & The American Dietetic Association, 1995.

MEAL PLANNING STRATEGIES, TIPS, & TECHNIQUES | WRITTEN BY: KRISTINE SINNER, MS, RDN

VARIETY, BALANCE, & MODERATION #HowToMealPlan

Visualizing Portion Sizes

Dairy 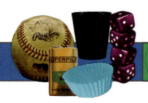   ### Vegetables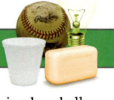

1 serving of cheese	is a 9-volt battery	1 serving of green salad	is a baseball
1 serving of milk	is a reg coffee cup	1 serving of baked potato	is a bar of soap
1 serving of ice cream	is a baseball	1 serving of tomato juice	is a small styrofoam cup
1 serving of cottage cheese	a cupcake wrapper	1 serving of cooked broccoli	is a standard light bulb
1 serving of kefir	is a shot glass	1 serving of asparagus	is 6 spears
		1 serving of baby carrots	is 7-8 carrots

Grains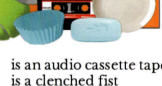

1 serving of potatoes	is a tennis ball	1 serving of bread	is an audio cassette tape
1 serving of pancake	is a music CD	1 serving of cereal	is a clenched fist
1 serving of cooked rice	is a cupcake wrapper	1 serving of cooked pasta	is a salad plate
1 serving of cornbread	is a small bar of soap		

Protein 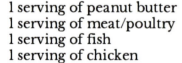   ### Fat

1 serving of peanut butter	is a ping-pong ball	1 serving of butter	is a thumb tip
1 serving of meat/poultry	is a deck of cards	1 serving of salad dressing	is a golf ball
1 serving of fish	is a checkbook	1 serving of avocado	is a pointer finger
1 serving of chicken	is a computer mouse	1 serving of liquid oil	is a poker chip
		1 serving of dark choc.	is a dental floss box
		1 serving of a brownie	is a makeup compact

Fruits 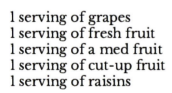   ### Snack Foods

1 serving of grapes	is a light bulb	1 serving of nuts	is 1 handful
1 serving of fresh fruit	is 7 cotton balls	1 serving of sm candies	is 1 handful
1 serving of a med fruit	is a tennis ball	chips/crackers/popcorn:	
1 serving of cut-up fruit	is a closed fist	1 serving	is 2 handfuls
1 serving of raisins	is a large egg	½ cup	is 1 man's handful
		⅓ cup	is 1 woman's handful

Serving Dishes/Utensils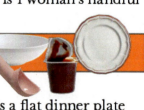

½ cup	is an ice-cream scoop	1 ½ cups pasta noodles	is a flat dinner plate
1 ½ cups	is a large soup bowl	½ cup pasta noodles	is a pudding cup

MEAL PLANNING STRATEGIES, TIPS, & TECHNIQUES | WRITTEN BY: KRISTINE SINNER, MS, RDN

VARIETY, BALANCE, & MODERATION   #HowToMealPlan

Portion Control Tips

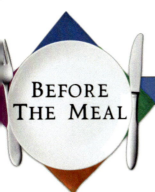
BEFORE THE MEAL

Practice pre-measuring food portions by using measuring cups and spoons until you feel comfortable visualizing approximate portion sizes.

Spend time familiarizing yourself with the everyday items you can associate with common foods you eat on the *"Visualizing Portion Sizes"* handout.

Read food labels on packaged foods and follow the indicated portion size for (1) serving. Keep in mind that occasionally the portion size indicated can actually be more than (1) serving.

Purchase foods that are pre-portioned, such as cottage cheese, yogurt, and snack sized dried fruits. These are great for on the go snacks as well as lunchboxes.

Portion foods for a single serving into a bowl or baggie versus eating out of the bag or box whenever possible.

Break down bulk items into single servings and store them in your pantry or refrigerator drawers and shelves to make them easy to grab when passing by or on the way out.

Keep a sufficient stock of ¼ cup, ½ cup, 1 cup, and 2 cups plastic food storage containers. The portion size is typically printed on the bottom of these containers and serve as a very useful tool for portion control when eating away from the home.

Whenever possible cook in large batches and freeze whatever portions you do not intend to consume right away.

DURING THE MEAL

Utilize '*the plate method*' by using a salad plate instead of a dinner plate for vegetables, protein, and grains. Then add a fruit and dairy to complete the meal.

Avoid eating directly out of containers or bags. Portion food out for single servings into a bowl or snack bag.

Avoid serving meals 'family style' and instead portion foods out onto your plate before sitting down to the table.

Use a juice cup instead of a tall tumbler cup when drinking calorie containing fluids.

Use a dinner spoon instead of a soup spoon.

Avoid distractions at meal time that can come from watching TV, scrolling on a smartphone, working on a computer, or reading to avoid overeating. Staying present when eating is important to note the taste and smell of food, as well as to key into hunger/fullness cues.

Eat slowly. Put the fork down between bites and thoroughly smell, chew, and taste your food.

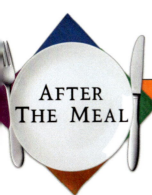
AFTER THE MEAL

Store leftovers in individual serving size containers versus one large container so you can take out only what you need at the next meal.

MEAL PLANNING STRATEGIES, TIPS, & TECHNIQUES | WRITTEN BY: KRISTINE SINNER, MS, RDN

VARIETY, BALANCE, & MODERATION

#HowToMealPlan

BREAKFAST IDEAS

1. Scrambled eggs or liquid egg whites/egg substitute with feta, spinach, tomatoes, peppers, and a mini toasted whole grain bagel
2. Spinach and eggs scrambled with salsa and diced avocado with a whole or sprouted grain tortilla
3. Cooked oats made with milk or vanilla milk substitute, protein powder, cinnamon, cocoa powder, flaxseeds, raisins, and chopped almonds, pecans or walnuts.
4. Vanilla or plain Greek yogurt with ancient grains granola, sliced raw almonds and blackberries
5. Protein shake made with 2 scoops of vanilla protein powder, any frozen fruit, ice, and water
6. Vanilla fortified instant breakfast pouch blended with half a frozen banana, frozen blueberries, flaxseed, wheat germ, and milk or milk substitute
7. Kefir with ancient grains granola
8. Scrambled eggs or egg substitute in the middle of a whole-wheat tortilla topped with salsa and shredded cheese
9. Hard boiled egg, whole wheat toast, margarine, and a bowl of fresh berries
10. Veggie, egg, and sausage sandwich: vegetarian sausage patty on a whole wheat English muffin with a slice of cheese and fruit
11. Scrambled eggs with diced peppers, onions, tomatoes, a pinch of shredded cheese, salsa, and whole wheat toast.
12. Hot wheat or oat bran cereal prepared with milk or milk substitute and a hard boiled egg
13. Omelet made with spinach, diced tomatoes, a pinch of mozzarella and a melon wedge.
14. Protein shake: 2 scoops of protein powder, water, ice, peanut butter, and ½ of a banana
15. Mashed avocado, eggs and spinach on whole or sprouted grain bread with everything bagel seasoning
16. Scrambled eggs, veggie sausage, whole grain toast, margarine, and juice.
17. Homemade trail mix: whole grain cereal squares, nuts, and dried fruit with a container of yogurt
18. Whole grain cereal topped with bananas and skim milk or milk substitute
19. Whole wheat waffle or pancake mix, liquid eggs added to batter, margarine, light syrup, veggie sausage, and orange juice.
20. 100% Whole grain waffle topped with natural peanut butter, a sprinkle of wheat germ, a drizzle of honey, and sliced banana
21. Canadian bacon, fried egg, and cheddar cheese on a toasted whole grain sandwich thin
22. Whole grain pancake or waffle batter with an added scoop of vanilla protein powder, pumpkin puree, cinnamon, vanilla extract, maple or agave syrup, margarine, a melon wedge, and a cup of milk
23. Whole grain cold cereal with skim milk and blueberries or strawberries
24. Toasted whole-wheat bagel topped with cottage cheese and fruit
25. Natural peanut butter whole wheat crackers or toast and a banana
26. Natural peanut butter on an apple dipped in wheat germ and topped with raisins

-25-

VARIETY, BALANCE, & MODERATION

#HowToMealPlan

LUNCH IDEAS

1. Almond butter and banana sandwich on whole grain bread with sliced bananas (try flavored almond butters such as chia seeds and cinnamon for flavorful variations).
2. Chicken and quinoa bowl with sweet potato, brussels sprouts, and dry roasted almonds
3. Tuna sandwich: whole grain bread, albacore tuna mixed with light mayo, pickle relish, lettuce, tomato slices, and an orange
4. Bean or meat chili with cornbread crackers
5. Greek chicken salad: romaine, tomato, red onion, feta cheese, red basil vinegar, Kalamata olives, and a whole grain pita
6. Whole grain English muffin pizza: tomato sauce, shredded mozzarella cheese, and veggie toppings as desired
7. Cottage cheese with mixed fruit and nut plate: melons, grapes, pineapple, pistachios, and whole grain crackers
8. Whole grain pizza crust or sandwich rounds with pesto, artichoke hearts, olives, roasted peppers, and cheese
9. Asian chicken wraps: chicken salad, red cabbage, edamame, and carrots in a spinach tortilla with sesame dressing
10. Cowboy caviar salad: corn, black bean, red onion, cilantro, avocado, and lime juice with corn tortilla chips
11. Pita pizza with any combo of mushrooms, peppers, olives, onion, pineapple, lean ham, turkey pepperoni, and mozzarella or parmesan cheese
12. Edamame pasta, tomatoes, halved cherry tomatoes, diced green peppers, feta cheese, garbanzo beans, parmesan cheese, and canola or olive oil-based vinaigrette dressing
13. Veggie burger on a whole grain roll with lettuce, tomato, slice cheese, pickles, mayo or avocado spread, and baked chips or pretzel sticks
14. Burrito bowl: cubed meat or tofu with black or pinto beans, brown rice, peppers, salsa, and guacamole
15. Chopped cobb salad- deli meat, egg whites, shredded cheese, lettuce, veggies as desired, and salad dressing
16. Caesar salad: Romaine, grilled shrimp or chicken, shredded parmesan cheese, croutons, and caesar dressing
17. Sliced grilled chicken with baked sweet potato and broccoli, cauliflower, carrots, or mixed vegetables
18. Mixed green salad with chopped chicken, chopped egg, granny smith apples, walnuts, and feta cheese
19. Kale salad with salmon or chicken, red cabbage, almonds, green apple, and lemon avocado dressing
20. Toasted peanut butter sandwich on whole grain bread with banana and carrot sticks
21. Broth based soup with a mixed greens salad, croutons, and a lite dressing
22. Whole wheat rotini pasta tossed with garbanzo beans, olive oil or pesto, halved cherry tomatoes, and grated Parmesan or Romano cheese
23. Stir-fry beef strips or marinated tofu with snow peas, water chestnuts, carrots, red bell peppers, brown rice, and fruit
24. Turkey burger on a whole grain sandwich round with red onion, tomato, lettuce, and avocado.
25. Bean burrito- refried or black beans in a tortilla with shredded cheese, lettuce, tomato, avocado, and salsa

VARIETY, BALANCE, & MODERATION

#HowToMealPlan

DINNER IDEAS

1. Asian chicken salad: fresh romaine lettuce, sliced red, yellow and green peppers, shredded carrots and red cabbage, red onion, diced grilled chicken, mandarin orange segments, spicy peanuts, sesame ginger dressing.

2. Broiled blackened salmon, bulgur pilaf, asparagus spears, and a fruit parfait (bowl of mixed berries with dollop of vanilla Greek yogurt)

3. Grilled chicken breast, rosemary/ garlic roasted red potato wedges, and fresh steamed broccoli

4. Whole grain pasta, ground meat or veggie crumbles, spaghetti sauce, shredded parmesan cheese, and a mixed green salad with 3-4 different colored veggies and salad dressing

5. Black (or other) bean soup with whole wheat or corn tortilla, shredded cheddar, and a dollop of plain Greek yogurt

6. Breakfast for dinner: protein whole grain pancakes with eggs and uncured turkey sausage links

7. Sliced roast turkey tenderloin, wild rice, and fresh cooked green beans

8. Lemon pepper shrimp with edamame or whole grain fettuccini noodles and sautéed spinach

9. Grilled steak, oven baked sweet potato with cottage cheese, cauliflower, and broccoli blend

10. Taco salad: ground turkey, chicken or beef, romaine lettuce, tomatoes, onions, diced green peppers, shredded cheese, black or kidney beans, cilantro, salsa, avocado, and baked tortilla chips.

11. Asian spinach salad: chopped rotisserie chicken (skinless), spinach, low fat feta, sliced red onion, chopped walnuts, mandarin oranges, ginger soy dressing, and sesame seeds.

12. Sausage and pepper stir fry: sliced grilled or sautéed chicken or turkey sausage with sautéed red, yellow, and green peppers & onions with quinoa

13. Shrimp and edamame pasta with pesto and pine nuts, spinach salad with strawberries and walnuts

14. Pork tenderloin chop + red potatoes and peas + applesauce

15. Ground turkey tacos/tostadas (whole grain or corn tortilla shells), shredded lettuce, shredded Monterey Jack or Cheddar, diced tomato, salsa, sour cream, sliced avocado

16. Steak kebabs: red, yellow or green peppers, new potatoes, onion, mushrooms + brown rice

17. Chicken stir fry: pea pods, carrots, water chestnuts, peppers, bamboo shoots, brown rice, and pineapple

18. Slow cooker beef pot roast with baby new potatoes, carrots, onions, and celery

19. Fish tacos on corn tortillas , black beans, and mango lime salsa

20. Veggie lasagna with a garden salad, whole wheat garlic roll, and a cluster of red or black grapes.

21. Slow cooker meatball, kale, bean, and barley soup with roll and side salad

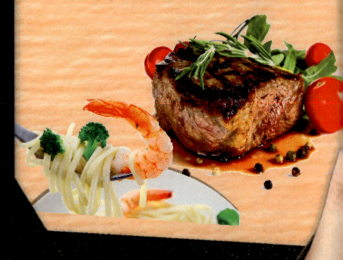

VARIETY, BALANCE, & MODERATION
#HowToMealPlan

SNACK IDEAS

1. Banana or apple w/ natural peanut butter
2. Any melon cubes w/ cottage cheese
3. Cucumber slices w/ veggie cream cheese on whole grain bread
4. Whole grain mini bagel w/ veggie cream cheese or flavored hummus
5. Honeydew melon w/ Greek yogurt
6. Red grape cluster w/ string cheese
7. Hard-boiled egg w/ bottled hot sauce
8. Ricotta cheese w/ cocoa powder
9. Apple, natural peanut butter, dried oats, raisins & honey
10. Red bell pepper strips w/ guacamole
11. Kale chips
12. Watermelon w/ pistachios & edamame
13. Sliced pears w/ ricotta cheese
14. Greek yogurt dip (vegetable soup mix blended w/ plain Greek yogurt) w/ fresh veggies or whole wheat pretzels to dip
15. Dark chocolate squares w/ walnut halves
16. Cantaloupe slices wrapped in prosciutto
17. Carrots w/ hummus & wheat crackers
18. Celery w/ natural peanut butter & raisins
19. Cheddar cheese w/ a pear or red apple
20. Coffee shop oatmeal & fruit w/ milk or milk sub latte
21. Refrigerated protein nut butter bar
22. Bottled protein shake or chocolate milk
23. Whole grain crackers w/ hummus, natural peanut butter, or reduced fat cheese
24. Whole grain crackers, pita, bread or bagel w/ hard-boiled egg salad
25. Whole grain cereal & milk or yogurt
26. Whole grain bread, bagel or English muffin w/ natural peanut butter
27. Whole grain bread, slice of cheese, & deli meat
28. Whole grain waffle, natural peanut butter & honey + sprinkle of wheat germ
29. Whole grain waffle w/ cup of milk
30. ½ egg salad sandwich & avocado
31. Whole grain tortilla + black bean dip
32. Whole grain pita + hummus
33. Whole grain tortilla, salsa, & cheese
34. Popcorn + parmesan cheese
35. Snack sized Kefir or drinkable yogurt
36. String cheese wrapped in deli meat & rolled in a whole grain tortilla
37. Rice cakes w/ ricotta cheese & salsa
38. Rice cakes w/ ricotta & cocoa powder
39. Rice cakes w/ natural peanut butter
40. Graham crackers & milk or yogurt
41. Graham crackers w/ natural peanut butter
42. Black bean dip & tortilla chips
43. Instant dehydrated soup cup (just add water) minestrone, split pea, black bean
44. Whole grain fig bar
45. Dried cherries & green peas w/ cashews
46. Chicken strips, cheese, soft taco w/ salsa

SECTION II
SHOPPING & COOKING

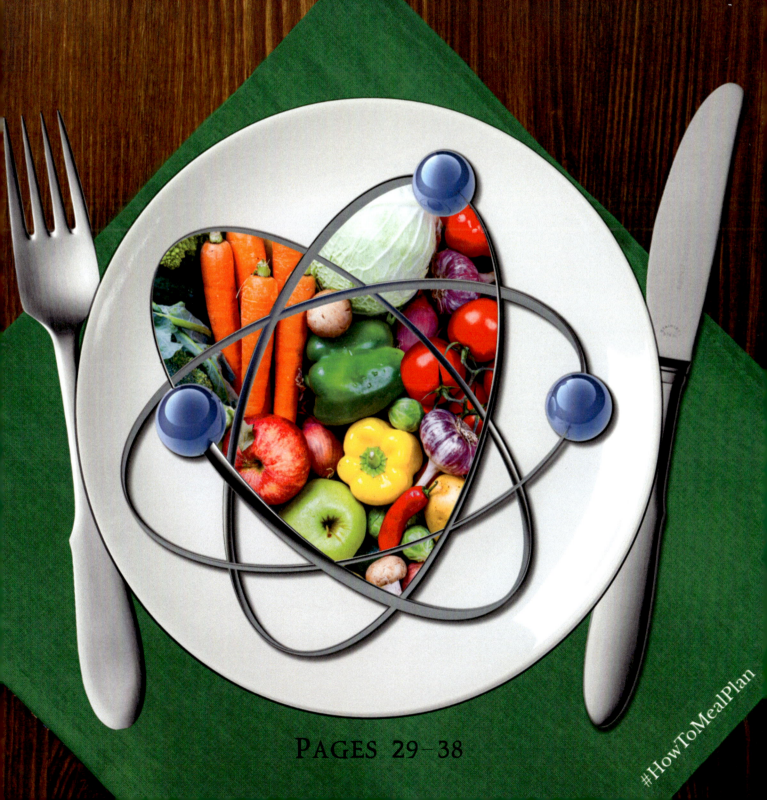

PAGES 29–38

SHOPPING & COOKING

#HowToMealPlan

Nutrition At The Grocery Store

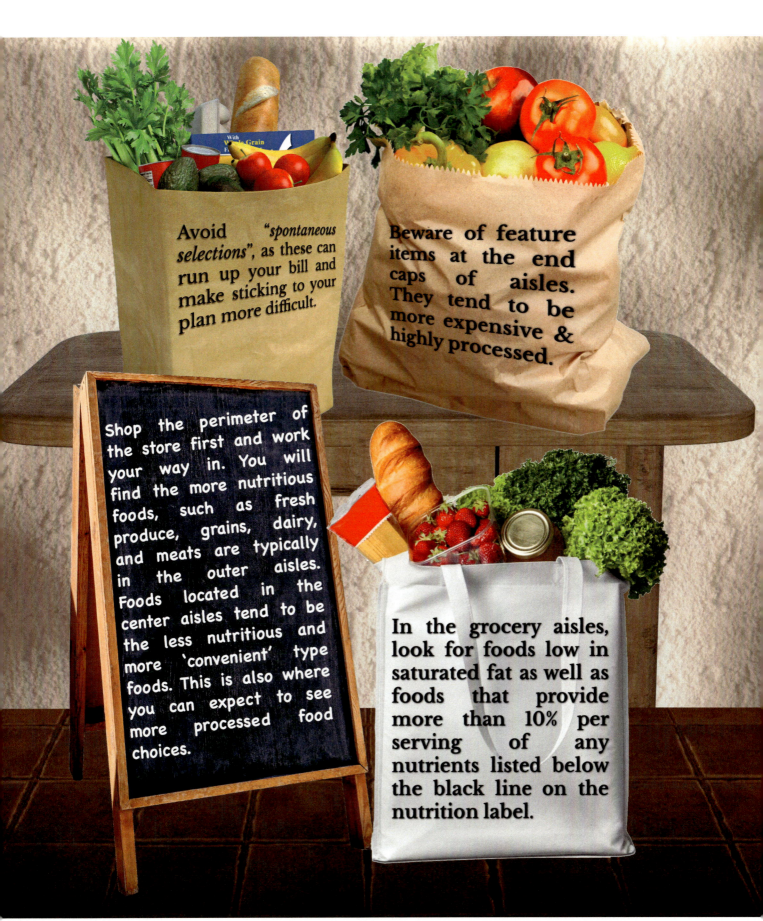

Avoid "*spontaneous selections*", as these can run up your bill and make sticking to your plan more difficult.

Beware of feature items at the end caps of aisles. They tend to be more expensive & highly processed.

Shop the perimeter of the store first and work your way in. You will find the more nutritious foods, such as fresh produce, grains, dairy, and meats are typically in the outer aisles. Foods located in the center aisles tend to be the less nutritious and more 'convenient' type foods. This is also where you can expect to see more processed food choices.

In the grocery aisles, look for foods low in saturated fat as well as foods that provide more than 10% per serving of any nutrients listed below the black line on the nutrition label.

MEAL PLANNING STRATEGIES, TIPS, & TECHNIQUES | WRITTEN BY: KRISTINE SINNER, MS, RDN

SHOPPING & COOKING

#HowToMealPlan

The 4 P's: Plan, Purchase, Prep, & Pack

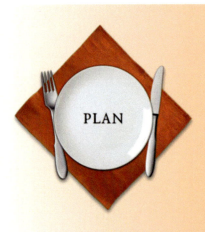

Invest in a durable and insulated lunch bag, a thermos for hot and cold foods, several plastic seal tight containers in various sizes, regular and snack size storage baggies, 2-3 refreezable blocks for a cooler, and a variety pack of disposable utensils. Find out what day the weekly ad for your local grocery store comes out, and get in a rhythm of checking current sales and coupons through their flyer or on the app. Keep this information in mind and scroll through your favorite recipe app to select 3 main meals to prepare for the week. Plan to prepare extra and use leftovers on days you won't be making something fresh and then create your shopping list. It's a good practice to keep a running inventory of what you already have on hand so when you run out of something you can add it to your list to pick up on your next trip to the grocery store.

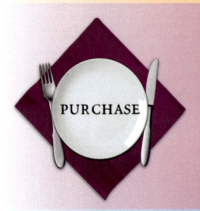

Stick to your list in order to avoid impulse purchases and endcap promotions. It is highly encouraged to shop after you have eaten so you are not hungry. This can also save you money because you will be far less likely to purchase more than you intended or maybe even afford. Shop early in the morning to take advantage of markdowns on fresh produce, meats, and dairy items. It's also a good idea to aim to go on days that are less busy, avoid weekends, and be sure to stock up on sale items of things you need. If grocery store anxiety fuels your impulse buys, consider ordering online and taking advantage of grocery store pick up or delivery services. This is also very useful for those with physical limitations, the elderly, caregivers, and of course busy parents.

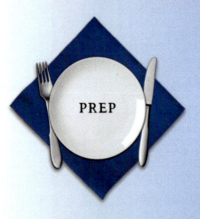

Pre-wash and cut whole fruits and vegetables into slices, wedges, sticks and quarters as soon as you get home from the store. Different shapes make food more interesting to eat and taking the time to do this will help you to stay interested in making better nutritious snack choices. Place prepped food at eye level in the fridge. For quick access to the more nutritious snack choices without needing too much thought, fill the bottom drawers with individual fruit, yogurt, pre-cut veggie bags, string cheese, juice boxes for kids, and so on. Display nuts and dried fruit in clear vacuum containers on your counter tops and be sure it is at eye level for quick snacks in passing. Also, at eye level, in your pantry place whole wheat or whole grain crackers, oatmeal cereal bites or bars, nuts, pretzels, and so on in seal tight containers or individually portioned baggies.

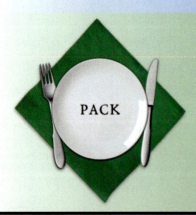

Prepare for the next day's meals and snacks the night before! Time is tight in the morning, and rushing through preparation often means compromising on nutrition or skipping prep time altogether in favor of vending machines and drive-through windows. Use your insulated lunch bag, thermos, and seal tight containers to pack your food. If you have perishable items to pack and take with you, be sure to use the re-freezable blocks in your insulated bag. Pack non perishable snacks to keep in the car or computer bag for long commutes and unexpected delays. This will prevent getting overly hungry and the urge for fast food, stopping at a convenience store, or bingeing when you get home.

MEAL PLANNING STRATEGIES, TIPS, & TECHNIQUES | WRITTEN BY: KRISTINE SINNER, MS, RDN

SHOPPING & COOKING

#HowToMealPlan

Grocery Store "Best Picks"

PRODUCE

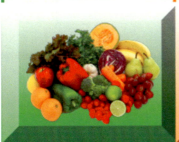

There are no foods in this category that do not make the '*best picks*' list.

Featured items that are currently in season will provide the best quality.

Choose a variety of deeply colored fruits & vegetables, the darkest of greens, the deepest of reds, the brightest of yellows & oranges, and the boldest of blues.

Go for organic when the food item has thin skin or when the skin is commonly eaten.

Over all, your best picks will be those items that present clean, firm, without foul odors, and void of any cuts, dents, soft spots, black spots, or damage.

OILS, FATS, & BAKING

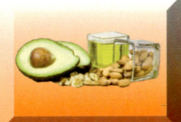

Omega-3 - Olive oil, Canola Oil

Omega-6 - Sunflower Oil, Safflower Oil, Corn Oil, Soybean Oil, Cottonseed Oil

Whether you chose butter or margarine is a matter of personal preference and both can be acceptable in moderate amounts.

Chopped Nuts, Seeds, Pumpkin Seeds, Wheat Germ, Pumpkin Puree, Dried Fruits, Dates

Ground Flax Meal, Flax Seeds, Chia Seeds, and Hemp Seeds

Whole Wheat Flour and Bread Crumbs

CANS & JARS

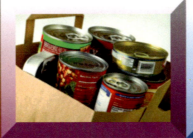

Any Legume - Peas, Lentils, Black, Kidney, White, Garbanzo, Pinto

Any Vegetable- Lower sodium varieties are available if you need to watch your salt intake

Any Fruits in Water or Light Syrups

Low Sodium Tomatoes and Tomato Paste/Reduced Sodium Bean, Pea or Lentil Based soups.

Chunk Albacore Tuna in Water/Canned Salmon

Peanut Butter- Natural, Cashew Butter, Almond Butter, Sunflower Butter

CEREAL

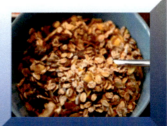

Choose High Fiber (>3 g/serving)

100% Whole Grain Oats- Plain or Low/No Added Sugar

Wheat Germ and Unprocessed Bran- easy to sprinkle on anything for extra nutritional boost

Instant breakfast pouches, available in several flavors and great as a smoothie base

Protein Powder

Oat based, Shredded Wheat Style, Fortified Cereals, Ancient Grains and Granola

MEAL PLANNING STRATEGIES, TIPS, & TECHNIQUES | WRITTEN BY: KRISTINE SINNER, MS, RDN

SHOPPING & COOKING

#HowToMealPlan

Grocery Store "Best Picks"

ETHNIC	BAKERY, BREADS, & CRACKERS	CONDIMENTS	DELI
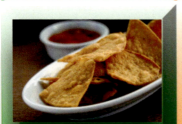	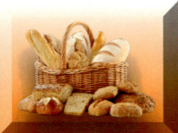	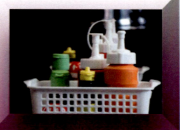	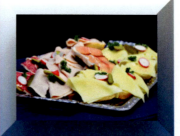
Corn and Whole Grain Tortillas Black Beans Jarred Black Bean or other Bean Dips Low-Fat or Vegetarian Refried Beans Canned Chilies/Spices Tomatoes	Look for grains with > 3g fiber/serving Choose 100% Whole Grain Breads, English Muffins, Tortillas, Pita, Flatbreads, Sandwich Thins, Rolls, and Buns. Crackers – look for those containing 2 or more grams of fiber/serving	Salsa, Hot Sauce Vinegar, Mustard Capers Bottled Marinades, Bottled Lemon and Lime Juice Jarred Red Peppers, Jarred Artichokes Olive or Canola Based Mayonnaise Lemon Pepper, Salt Free Seasonings	Natural Reduced Sodium Lean Meats Low Fat Cheeses Heart Healthy Labels *Deli meats can be ordered sliced thin or in thick slices (1-2 " thick), which makes great cubes to use for snacks or meals

MEAL PLANNING STRATEGIES, TIPS, & TECHNIQUES | WRITTEN BY: KRISTINE SINNER, MS, RDN

SHOPPING & COOKING

#HowToMealPlan

Grocery Store "Best Picks"

FROZEN	MEAT & SEAFOOD	PASTA, RICE, GRAINS, DRIED BEANS	SNACKS & NUTS
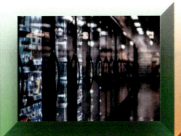	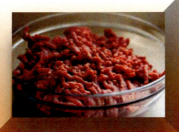	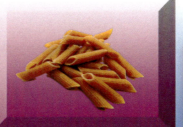	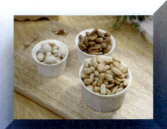
All Vegetables, Plain or Mixed All Fruits- Berries (great for smoothies), Mangoes, Pineapple, Cherries, Peaches Whole Grain Waffles Grilled or Baked Fish/Shrimp 100% Frozen Fruit Bars, High Protein Ice Cream and Bars Veggie Burgers/Turkey Burgers	Coldwater Fish Contains the Highest Levels of EPA and DHA Salmon, Mackerel, Tuna, Sturgeon Shrimp, and Anchovies 1½ ounces Fish Has 1 Gram Omega-3. Boneless Skinless Chicken Breast, Lean Ground Beef, Turkey and Chicken Beef : Round, Sirloin, Venison, Bison Pork Tenderloin - Well Trimmed	Bulgur. Quinoa, Couscous, Farro, Barley Rice- Brown, Red, Black White, Jasmine Legumes: Kidney Beans, Black Beans, Great Northern, Garbanzo, Lentils, Split Peas Pasta- Whole Grain, Wheat, Edamame, Chick Pea, Red Lentil, Black Bean	Raw Unsalted Nuts Almonds, Walnuts, Pistachios, Cashews Popcorn, Flavored or Plain Varieties Dried Green Peas Granola, Checkered Cereal Bites Whole Wheat Pretzels, Woven Wheat Crackers, or Super Seed Rounds Fig Bars, Whole Grain Oat & Dried Fruit Cookies, Dark Chocolate

MEAL PLANNING STRATEGIES, TIPS, & TECHNIQUES | WRITTEN BY: KRISTINE SINNER, MS, RDN

SHOPPING & COOKING

#HowToMealPlan

Grocery Store "Best Picks"

BEVERAGES	JUICE & EGGS	MISC	MILK, CHEESE, & YOGURT
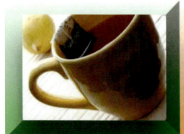	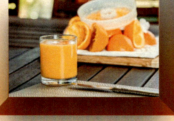	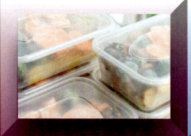	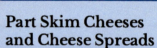
Milk, Water, Fruit Juice- Unsweetened, Low Sodium Vegetable Juice	Fortified 100% Unsweetened Juices with Pulp- Orange, Grapefruit	Protein Bars and Protein Powder	Part Skim Cheeses and Cheese Spreads
Seltzer or Carbonated Water	Fruit and Protein Smoothie Blends	Whole Wheat Pizza Crust	Low-Fat Shredded Cheese Varieties or Chunk Cheeses
Flavored Fortified Water	Pomegranate and Tart Cherry Juices	Storage bags - Sandwich and Snack Size	Low-Fat Plain or Greek Yogurt
Herbal Tea/Coffee	Raw Eggs In the Carton and Pre-Hard Boiled Eggs	Re-sealable Containers in Various sizes (1⁄4 cup – 3 cup sizes)	Low-Fat Sour Cream
	Liquid Eggs in Carton and Egg Substitute	Steam Bags, Insulated Lunch Bag, & Freezer Packs	Low-Fat Cottage Cheese, Ricotta Cheese
			Kefir

Meal Planning Strategies, Tips, & Techniques | Written By: Kristine Sinner, MS, RDN

SHOPPING & COOKING

#HowToMealPlan

Nutritious Pantry Basics

Whole grain waffle and pancake mix

Cereals: rolled oats, oatmeal, muesli, ancient grains, fiber rich fortified hot and cold cereals

Canned Legumes: dried peas, whole or refried beans, lentils

Canned fruit, dried fruit, and raisins

Natural nut butters in jars, pouches, spreads or powdered form

Baked corn tortilla strips, chips, or shells

Meats/Fish: cans or pouches of salmon, albacore tuna, and chicken breast

Canned Vegetables: tomato paste, corn, peas, green beans, pumpkin puree, canned chilies

Grains: single rice varieties (*brown, white, black and red*), pouches of mixed grain varieties, quinoa, farro, bulgur, barley, couscous, whole grain pasta varieties, edamame, lentil, chickpeas, black beans

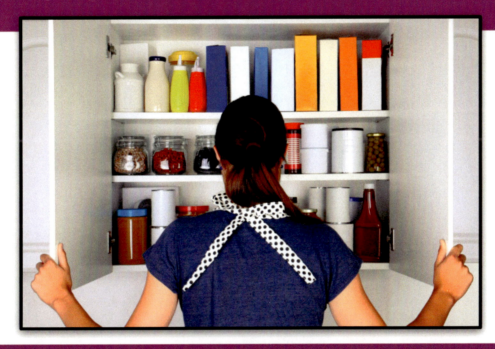

Cereal Bars: oat, ancient grain, fruit and nut

Protein bars and cookies

Complete instant breakfast pouches

Low-sodium bean or legume soups

Fortified whole grain instant cold and hot cereals

Fig cookies and bars

Liquid flavoring extracts (vanilla, almond, pecan, chocolate, mint)

Pretzels, whole wheat or multigrain crackers, super seed crackers, rice or popcorn cakes

Protein Powder (*there are varieties to accommodate tolerances & preferences*)

Honey, agave syrup, marmalade, superfruit berry sauce, real maple syrup

Spices for flavoring baked goods and smoothies (*cinnamon, nutmeg, allspice, etc...*) and for meals (*garlic powder, lemon pepper, italian blend, etc...*)

Jarred salsa, sun-dried tomatoes, olives, black bean dip, marinara, vinegar, and oils

SHOPPING & COOKING

#HowToMealPlan

Nutritious Countertop Basics

"If you see it, you just might eat it!"

Nuts (*pistachios, walnuts, almonds, cashews*) displayed in clear seal tight jars as a visual reminder

Dried Fruits: cranberries, blueberries, apricots, apple rings, raisins, mangoes, and dates (*display in a clear seal-tight jars as visual reminders to grab when in need of a quick snack*)

Whole Fruit: Fill a fruit bowl with bananas, apples, oranges, peaches, pears or other seasonal varieties of your liking

Prepare a countertop basket that contains onions, potatoes, and heads of garlic (*this is a great way to remember to use these items during the week*)

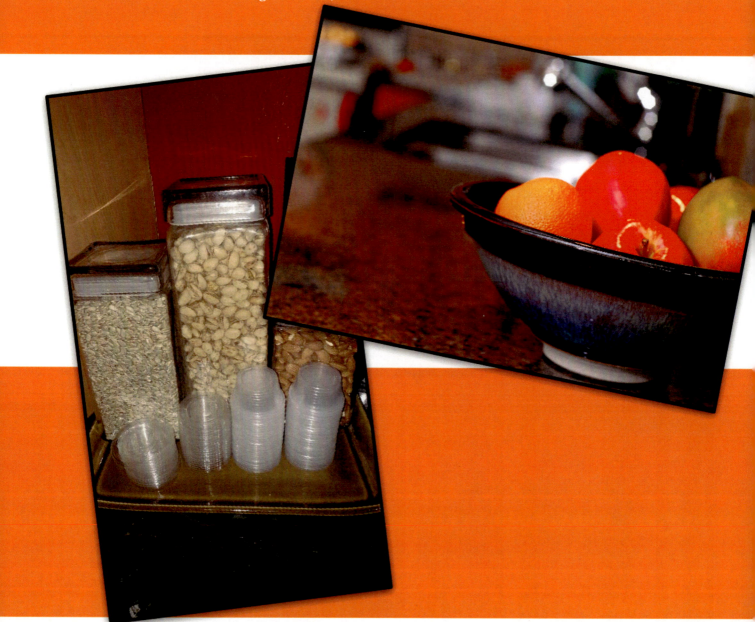

Meal Planning Strategies, Tips, & Techniques | Written By: Kristine Sinner, MS, RDN

SHOPPING & COOKING

#HowToMealPlan

Nutritious Refrigerator Basics

Dairy: milk, yogurt, kefir, cottage cheese

Fortified Juice- orange, grapefruit, tart cherry, pomegranate.

Bottled Juice: lemon and lime juice

A Rainbow of Produce: reds (*bell peppers, tomatoes, apples*), orange (*oranges, cantaloupe, carrots*), yellows (*lemons, yellow peppers, squash*), purples (*grapes, blueberries, cabbage*), and green (*peppers, broccoli, kale, asparagus, brussels sprouts*)

Grains: whole/multi grain bread, sandwich thins, bagels, bagel thins, pitas, tortillas, english muffins.

Meats: sliced or cubed deli meats

Raw eggs, liquid and/or hard boiled

Real fruit spreads

Non-fat or low-fat milk, cheese slices, string or block cheese, cottage cheese, and yogurt

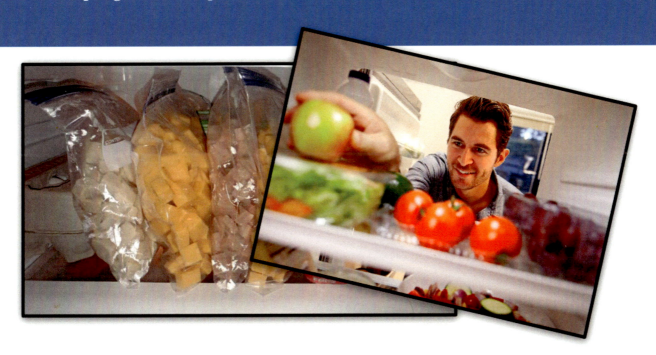

Misc: pesto, dijon mustard, balsamic vinegar, salad dressing, horseradish, capers, salsa, chopped jarred garlic, wheat germ, flaxseeds, hemp seeds and chia seeds

Fats and Oils: butter, canola or olive oil based margarine, olive oil mayo, and pesto

Dips & Spreads: hummus, avocado, jarred bean dip, 32oz. tub of plain Greek yogurt for making smoothies or as a sour cream substitute

Fresh herbs, squeeze tubed spices, and garlic

Meal Planning Strategies, Tips, & Techniques | Written By: Kristine Sinner, MS, RDN

SHOPPING & COOKING
Nutritious Freezer Basics

#HowToMealPlan

Uncured sausage/bacon - turkey, vegetarian, veggie meat crumbles

Individually wrapped quick frozen fish fillets- *Wild Salmon, Mahi Mahi, Cod, Halibut, Tuna, Sea Bass*

Frozen meats- *whole, breast, tenderloins, ground, patties, meatballs, meatless versions*

Microwavable whole grain turkey sausage, egg white, and cheese breakfast sandwiches

Microwaveable oatmeal bowls and fruit, super seed and ancient grains power bowls

Microwavable veggie medleys- *root veggies, barley and legume bowls, power bowls*

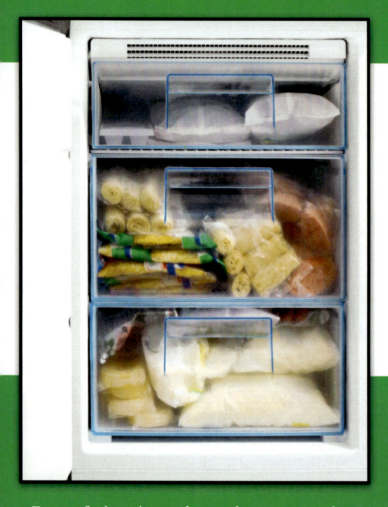

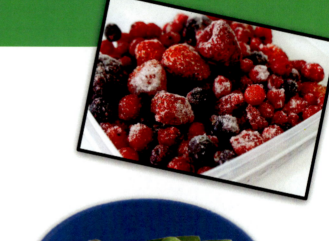

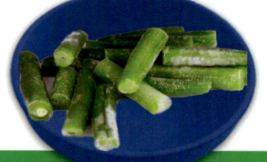

Whole grain waffles, pancakes, muffins, sprouted or seeded breads

Mixed frozen fruit and vegetable blends, great for smoothies

Frozen fruits- pineapple, peaches, mangoes, bananas, berries, and cherries

Buy fresh blueberries, blackberries, and raspberries in season and then freeze to enjoy later

Frozen fortified fruit juice concentrates

Shredded or chunk coconut

MEAL PLANNING STRATEGIES, TIPS, & TECHNIQUES | WRITTEN BY: KRISTINE SINNER, MS, RDN

SECTION III
Eating Away From Home

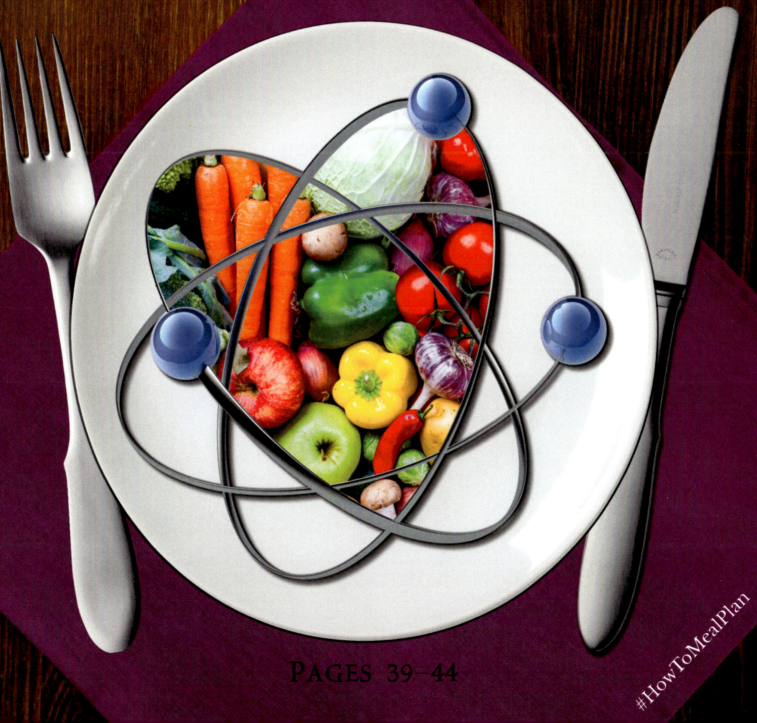

Pages 39–44

#HowToMealPlan

EATING AWAY FROM HOME

#HowToMealPlan

Restaurant Eating Tips & Suggestions

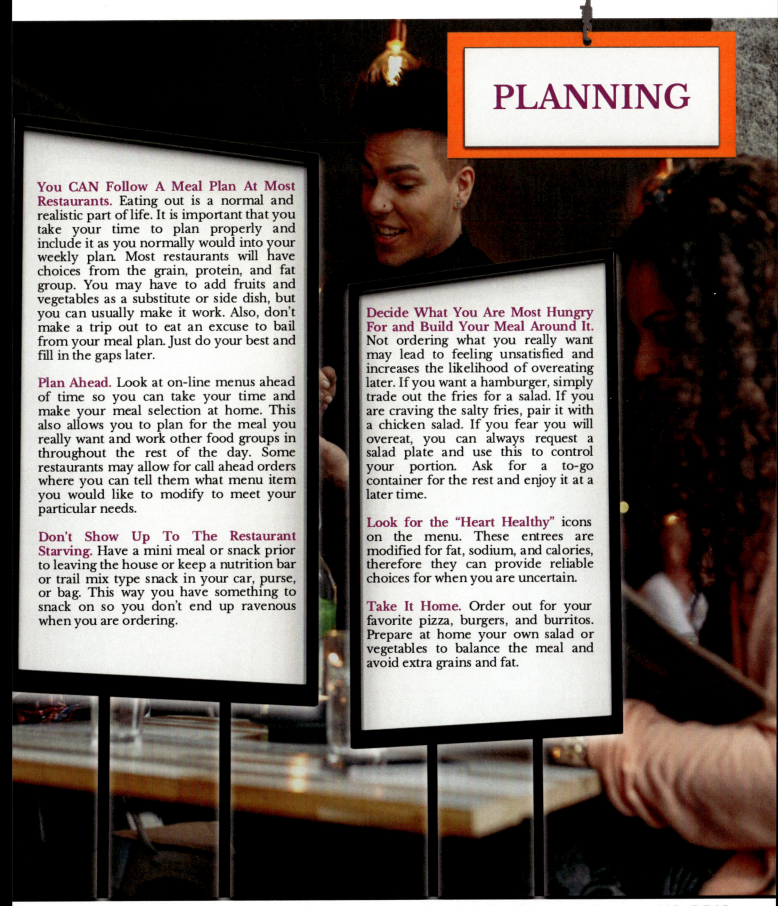

PLANNING

You CAN Follow A Meal Plan At Most Restaurants. Eating out is a normal and realistic part of life. It is important that you take your time to plan properly and include it as you normally would into your weekly plan. Most restaurants will have choices from the grain, protein, and fat group. You may have to add fruits and vegetables as a substitute or side dish, but you can usually make it work. Also, don't make a trip out to eat an excuse to bail from your meal plan. Just do your best and fill in the gaps later.

Plan Ahead. Look at on-line menus ahead of time so you can take your time and make your meal selection at home. This also allows you to plan for the meal you really want and work other food groups in throughout the rest of the day. Some restaurants may allow for call ahead orders where you can tell them what menu item you would like to modify to meet your particular needs.

Don't Show Up To The Restaurant Starving. Have a mini meal or snack prior to leaving the house or keep a nutrition bar or trail mix type snack in your car, purse, or bag. This way you have something to snack on so you don't end up ravenous when you are ordering.

Decide What You Are Most Hungry For and Build Your Meal Around It. Not ordering what you really want may lead to feeling unsatisfied and increases the likelihood of overeating later. If you want a hamburger, simply trade out the fries for a salad. If you are craving the salty fries, pair it with a chicken salad. If you fear you will overeat, you can always request a salad plate and use this to control your portion. Ask for a to-go container for the rest and enjoy it at a later time.

Look for the "Heart Healthy" icons on the menu. These entrees are modified for fat, sodium, and calories, therefore they can provide reliable choices for when you are uncertain.

Take It Home. Order out for your favorite pizza, burgers, and burritos. Prepare at home your own salad or vegetables to balance the meal and avoid extra grains and fat.

MEAL PLANNING STRATEGIES, TIPS, & TECHNIQUES | WRITTEN BY: KRISTINE SINNER, MS, RDN

EATING AWAY FROM HOME

Restaurant Eating Tips & Suggestions

PORTION CONTROL

Be mindful of the chip/breadbasket. Restaurants often provide these "eat as much as you want" goodies as you are pondering the menu. Be cautious of mindless noshing. This can contribute a considerable amount of fat and calories to your meal. If you choose to have the bread or chips on the table realize you may want to trade that out for a grain in your meal. Ask yourself, would you rather have the bread, chips or the fresh pasta?

Order from the kids or the appetizer menu. Most kid's meals and appetizers are served in realistic portions.

Restaurants don't determine your portion size, you do. Restaurants have standard portion sizes which are often served on platters or large dinner plates, most of which are double what the average person would need. Instead, request that the server bring you out a salad plate to portion your food onto, or have him box up half of your meal before it is brought out to you. It can be more economical to share a single entrée with a friend,

Avoid being seduced by more for your money deals. Buffets, super sizing and all you can eat gimmicks may save money in your wallet now, but you will pay with your health later. Watch out for terms such as super size, deluxe, jumbo. These items can contribute up to more than half of your daily needs for calories, fat and sodium!

EATING AWAY FROM HOME

#HowToMealPlan

Restaurant Eating Tips & Suggestions

PRACTICALITY

Preparation Methods. Look for terms such as: baked, broiled, boiled, roasted, grilled, and steamed, Avoid fried or sautéed and request foods served "**plain**" whenever possible.

Ask For Sides. Request for salad dressings, sauces, and gravies to be served on the side. Dip fork tines into low fat salad dressing and then the salad vs. pouring dressings over the entire salad.

Modify- It's OK! Swap out white bread for whole wheat, white rice for brown, cooked veggies for fresh, french fries for a plain baked potato, egg whites for regular eggs, spinach or romaine for iceberg lettuce, etc... Most restaurants are prepared and more than willing to accommodate.

Add If You Like! Request additional veggies on your sandwich or omelet or some legumes on your salad.

Eat Slower. Slow down the pace of your eating. Pay closer attention to how the food tastes, the texture, temperature, and mouth feel. This will make it easier to know when you are satisfied and avoid eating to the point of fullness (which is technically overeating).

Drink Water. Order water or milk instead of regular sodas. If you need something fizzy get seltzer water with lime. Sodas, juices and alcoholic beverages can add 200-400 kcals and do not provide any nutritional value.

Limit Alcoholic Beverages To One Serving. Alcoholic beverages oz. per oz. can pack a caloric punch and can also contribute to mindless overeating behaviors.

Stay Present. Enjoy your company while being mindful of your plate and fullness level.

Eat Your "Trigger" or Unsafe Foods In A Safe Place and/or Safe People. Rather than keep an entire batch of brownies at home, go out for a dessert with a friend you can trust to help you with your portions, or order and eat the item in a place where you will be less likely to overeat. Share a dessert with others at the table so you can try new and fun dishes without feeling like you have overdone it.

MEAL PLANNING STRATEGIES, TIPS, & TECHNIQUES | WRITTEN BY: KRISTINE SINNER, MS, RDN

EATING AWAY FROM HOME

#HowToMealPlan

Holidays, Vacations, & Special Occasions

Many people prepare for holidays, vacations, and special occasions with an expectation to overeat. While it may be tempting to do this in these situations, it is not a habit that you want to form. Enjoying special desserts and savory dishes however, is absolutely encouraged and when done alongside the tips listed below it can quite a satisfying experience.

BRING YOUR OWN FRUITS & VEGETABLES!

Even if the host is serving deep fried turkey, when you bring a fresh salad or fruit to the party you will ensure to have the balance needed in your meal. Snack on the foods you bring as appetizers so you are not starving when it's time for the main meal. This is also an extremely helpful tactic when on vacation as well. In addition to packing fruits and vegetables, be sure to also have a few protein sources to throw in a cooler or the refrigerator in your hotel room. This will make snacking and balancing meals so much easier. It is also helpful to keep protein bars and single serving baggies of trail mix in your purse or bag to avoid having only less desirable choices.

WORK IN PHYSICAL ACTIVITY!

Choose walking tours on vacation instead of bus tours. While you may not be able to do your exact workout routine, adding in physical activity can be very effective. On holidays make it a tradition to go for a walk or play a family game of basketball or tennis. If it is winter time go skiing or sledding!

BE WILLING TO THROW FOOD AWAY!

Even when times are tough, eating the rest of the mashed potatoes to the point of being stuffed is not going to save a lot of money in the long run. In fact, the risk to your health from doing this regularly can prove to be being far more expensive than any food you choose to throw away. Avoid the urge to eat the whole meal because someone else made it or you paid a higher price for it.

DO NOT "SAVE UP"!

The worst thing you can do is skip breakfast and lunch so that you can allow yourself to indulge in a huge Thanksgiving Feast. Instead, eat normal meals leading up to or around the holiday meal to ensure you are not starving when it's time to eat. The same rationale applies for vacations. Do not starve yourself the weeks before a vacation or cruise so you can overeat when you get there.

DO HAVE DESERT!

However, be a dessert snob! Often times we eat desserts because they are there and we haven't had it or allowed ourselves to have it in a while. Choose only desserts that you truly enjoy and listen to your bodies natural cue to stop. You may not be able to have Grandma's pumpkin pie every day, but you will have pie again and when that happens you will enjoy it so much more.

DON'T GIVE IN TO PRESSURE!

While your Grandma may be a little hurt when you don't accept seconds of her rice pudding, when you set appropriate boundaries it can end up being a non-issue. Boundaries can also be helpful on vacation when your friends or family are ordering more drinks or dessert when you are not in need of either. So, ask Grandma for a take home box, thank her for all the care and effort she put into the preparation, and know that's what she probably wants anyways.

MEAL PLANNING STRATEGIES, TIPS, & TECHNIQUES | WRITTEN BY: KRISTINE SINNER, MS, RDN

EATING AWAY FROM HOME

#HowToMealPlan

What to Bring or Make on Holidays

VOLUNTEER TO BRING OR MAKE THE FOLLOWING ON HOLIDAYS:

Artisan cheese and meat board with dried fruits, raw almonds, and cashews

Raw vegetables with savory yogurt veggie dip

Breads and Oils: seasoned, flavor infused olive oils and vinegars with shredded parmesan, ground black pepper, and some Artisan Crusty Bread

Fresh fruit bowl with a fruit dip

Deviled eggs

Hummus with seasoned olives, sliced cucumbers, and carrots

Ceviche: seafood, avocado, onion, and cilantro with lemon and lime

Caprese Salad: mozzarella, fresh basil, and sliced tomatoes with a balsamic vinegar glaze

Turkey, chicken, or lean ham and cheese roll ups

Fresh Greek, Pear, or Spring Salad

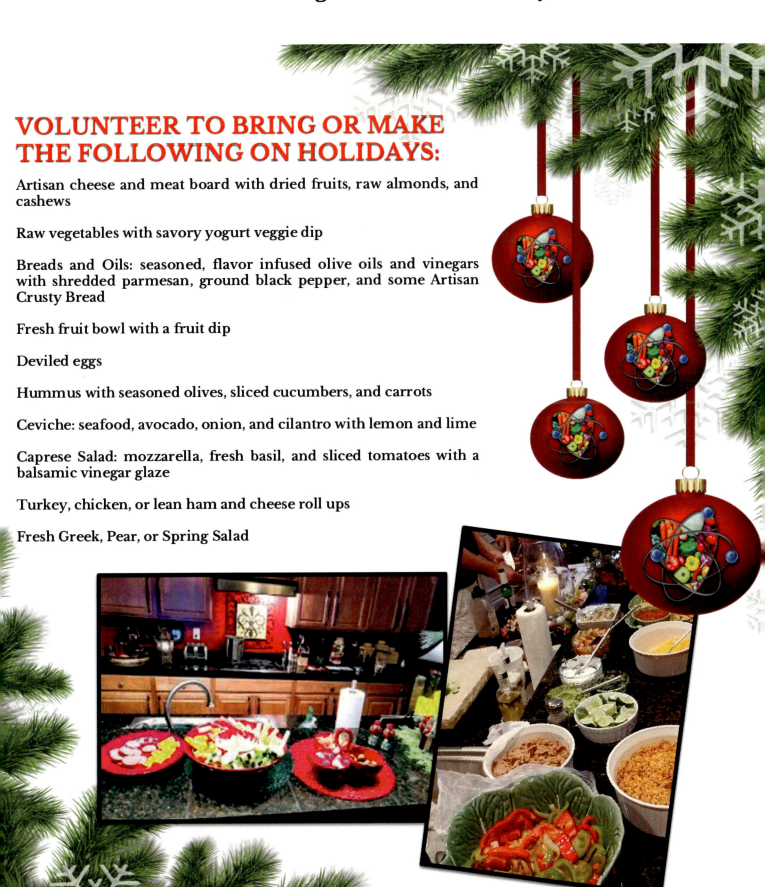

Meal Planning Strategies, Tips, & Techniques | Written By: Kristine Sinner, MS, RDN

EATING AWAY FROM HOME

#HowToMealPlan

Foods To Bring on Vacation

Keep protein bars and trail mix in your purse or bag to avoid having only less favorable options to choose from while away.

Travel with your own fruit, a few vegetable options, and some quick protein sources. If needed you can store it all in a cooler or your hotel fridge.

Doing this will make snacking and balancing meals while on vacation and also when away from home so much easier and far less stressful.

Trail mix-dried fruit and nuts
Breakfast cereal and or packaged oatmeal
Protein bars
Fresh fruit and veggies if possible

Jar of peanut butter
9 Grain crackers
Powdered Instant breakfast
Meat or turkey jerky

MEAL PLAN   MS, RDN

-44-

SECTION IV
Putting It All Together

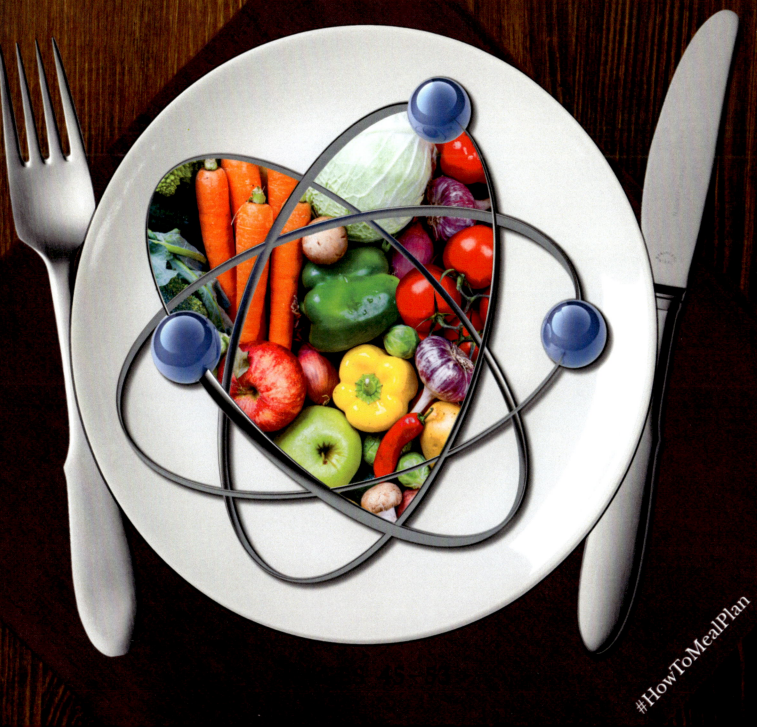

PUTTING IT ALL TOGETHER

#HowToMealPlan

How To Get Started

Step 1: Identify 1 dedicated hour every week for *Planning*

Step 2: Select a day & time every week for *Shopping*

Step 3: Decide on a day of the week for *Prepping*

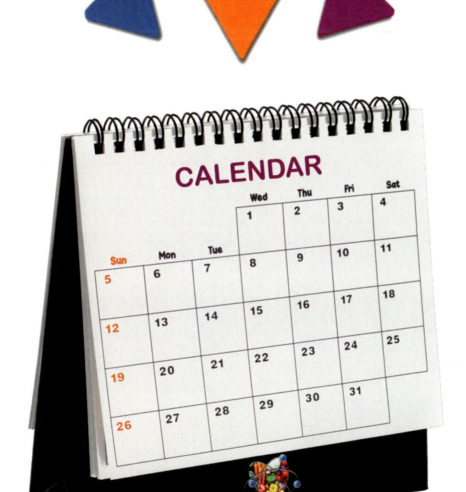

MEAL PLANNING STRATEGIES, TIPS, & TECHNIQUES | WRITTEN BY: KRISTINE SINNER, MS, RDN

PUTTING IT ALL TOGETHER

#HowToMealPlan

Planning For A Busy Week

Breakfasts: M, T, W, & Th will need to be something quick and simple to have on the way to work, and on Friday I will plan to go to the cafe drive thru and have a more substantial breakfast since it will be difficult to have a real lunch with my meeting and teleconference.

Lunches: T & W I can do whatever since there is nothing scheduled around lunch time. Th & F on the other hand will need to be super simple since I will be in the car one day and in meetings on the other. Probably bring a sandwich both days.

Snacks: With so much running around this week I will just make sure I have at least 2 non-perishable snacks in my purse each day, like trail mix or a protein bar. I will also bring some fresh fruit to keep in the fridge at the office so I can grab it if I need something extra to get me by.

Dinners: There really isn't much time to cook during the week so I am going to make a crockpot meal on Sunday so we will have leftovers on Monday night. Wednesday I will have a frozen home cooked meal from batch cooking last week. Tuesday & Thursday will be a pre-cooked meal from the store we can throw in the oven and Friday we will get the kids a pizza before Date Night!

MEAL PLANNING STRATEGIES & TECHNIQUES WRITTEN BY KRI SINNER, MS, RDN

PUTTING IT ALL TOGETHER

#HowToMealPlan

The Dedicated Planning Hour

Identify 1 day of the week to sit down for a Dedicated Planning Hour. Use this time to make your plan for the following 7 days. Follow the following steps every week, on the same day if possible, to create a good habit.

Step 1:

Prepare a *Master Inventory List** of what you currently have in your fridge, freezer, pantry, cupboards, and drawers. The first time you do this will take a little extra time since you are creating it. After it's finished, updating it each week will be quick and easy.

Step 2:

Peruse recipe books and do internet searches for recipes that sound appealing to you. Download your favorite recipe app and when you have free time 'favorite' the ones you might want to try so when you are doing your planning you can select one or two at a time. If you prefer a more traditional route, print the ones you like and use sticky notes to mark the page in your recipe book.

Step 3:

Plan all of the meals you need for the week during this dedicated planning hour so it's done and you can plan accordingly. Use the weekly meal planning template titled, *What I Plan To Eat This Week**. It will provide easy visualization of how the week is going to look as it relates to meal planning. It is a good practice to simultaneously have your calendar for the week open and ask yourself the following question:

> *Based on what is going on this week and when I will be home vs. out of the house, is this a week when batch cooking is needed in order to have leftovers available when time will not permit cooking and/or enough to freeze and store for another week's menu?*

If you are planning meals for you and your family, consider having theme nights, such as *Taco Tuesday* or *Sunday Steak Night*. Be sure to vary the items from week to week, and make it a point to try new recipes until you have created a considerable selection. It can be helpful to print out and keep them in a tabbed binder or electronically bookmark recipes that go over well for future reference. Include comments on each recipe so you don't have to rely on memory for things like if the meal tasted good, if it needed more flavor, or maybe it was was just....Eh!

Cross check the ingredients needed to prepare each recipe with your master inventory list for items you may already have. Using the *Grocery List Template**, add the items you don't have to your list so you are sure to get it when you are at the store.

*Forms & handouts referenced can be found in the appendix

MEAL PLANNING STRATEGIES, TIPS, & TECHNIQUES | WRITTEN BY: KRISTINE SINNER, MS, RDN

PUTTING IT ALL TOGETHER
#HowToMealPlan

Shopping Day

Step 1: Sales & Coupons

There are now several convenient ways to food shop, both online as well as by going directly to the grocery store. Create an online account for your favorite stores to stay informed of their latest sales and special promotions. Most stores have an app you can download as well, so to make things even easier remember to turn on notifications. 🔔

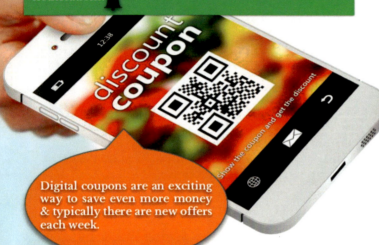

Digital coupons are an exciting way to save even more money & typically there are new offers each week.

Step 2: Go Shopping

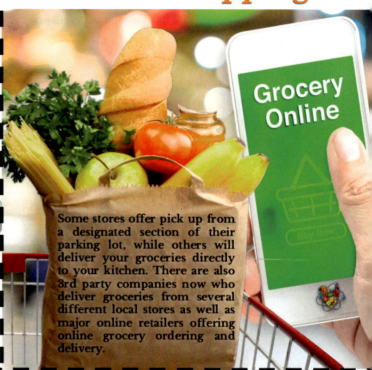

Some stores offer pick up from a designated section of their parking lot, while others will deliver your groceries directly to your kitchen. There are also 3rd party companies now who deliver groceries from several different local stores as well as major online retailers offering online grocery ordering and delivery.

Step 3: Organize Your Groceries

Organize your groceries when you get home so you are less likely to forget about items you've purchased which could deviate you from your plan. Items that come in larger boxes or containers such as nuts, strawberries, baby carrots, etc... can be broken down into convenient single servings using plastic baggies or containers and placed in the fridge, pantry or freezer right away. This allows for quick grab and go and helps to maintain a single serving consumption vs. eating directly from a container where it is quite easy to eat more than your body really wants.

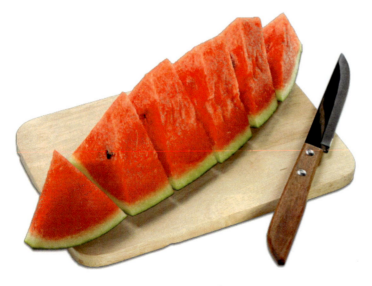

Tips To Get Started:

Cut up the your fruits and vegetables, such as a whole watermelon, as soon as you return home from the store. Portion it out into single serve baggies and store at eye level in the fridge so you can see it vs leaving it on the counter to get to it later. **The reality for most of us is that fresh foods often will go bad because we don't find the time to cut it up and properly store it.**

Use the entire bottom drawer of the fridge to store quick grab-and-go single serving items.

Meal Planning Strategies, Tips, & Techniques | Written By: Kristine Sinner, MS, RDN

PUTTING IT ALL TOGETHER

#HowToMealPlan

Prepping Your Weekly Staples

This list is an example of what a single person or a family could prepare to keep on-hand for the week. All items can be stored as single servings in individual plastic baggies or all together in one large plastic baggie. Be sure to place it at *eye level* in the fridge so you are guaranteed to see it. Whether the goal is to stock your quick snacks or batch cook and freeze, doing the actual portioning and cooking on this specific day will make choosing better food choices considerably easier.

Hard Boiled Eggs

Mixed Bean Salad

Roasted Potatoes

Whole Grain Pasta Spirals or Penne

Rice and Whole Grains

Hummus or Avocado Spread

Legumes and lentils

Overnight oats

Whole or Ground Beef, Turkey, Pork, Chicken or Fish. *Prepare it Baked, Broiled or Grilled*

Roasted Vegetables, Potatoes, Brussel Sprouts, Whole tomato, and Root Vegetables

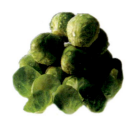 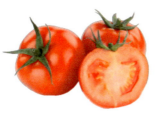 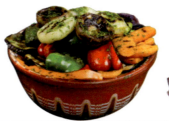 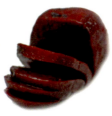 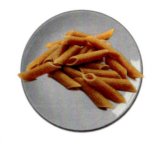 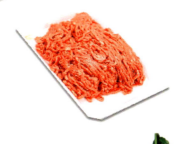

MEAL PLANNING STRATEGIES, TIPS, & TECHNIQUES | WRITTEN BY: KRISTINE SINNER, MS, RDN

PUTTING IT ALL TOGETHER

#HowToMealPlan

Organizing Your Groceries For Optimal Usage

1. Over-The-Door Plastic Shoe Holders
Store items like taco seasoning packets, fruit snacks, veggie dip, marinade pouches, etc...

2. Snack Bins
Clear the bottom shelf of the pantry for easy to reach snacking for kids.

3. Refrigerator Soda Pack
Used for storing canned goods such as veggies, beans, soups, fruit, etc... Decorate it to make a fun DIY project!

4. Small Mesh Laundry Bags
Store your fresh onions and garlic and then hang the bag on the back of a door or some open and convenient wall space using a nail or hooks.

5. Spice Drawer
Use a long drawer to hold spices. No more standing on tippy toes to find what you need.

6. Pants Hanger or Chip Clip
To hold bags of tortilla chips, pretzels, or any other similar bagged item. Clothespins make great bag closers as well.

7. Large Glass Jars With Scoops
For bulk items like what you can use the Mason Jars for, except here it would be when you have a larger quantity to store.

8. Souffle Cups With Lids
3-4 oz cups used to portion foods like hummus into single servings for easy grab & go options.

9. Bento Boxes & Plastic Containers With Lids
Use these to store leftover casseroles, ground taco meat, soups, etc...

10. Disposable Containers With Paper Lid
For leftovers that need to be dated or have specific instructions because you can write on the paper lid.

11. Plastic Baggies (small, large, and snack size)
Plastic baggies can be used for anything. They are great for storage and especially for portioned single serving snacks like trail mix or fruit.

12. Small & Large Muffin Tins With Paper Liners
Easy way to portion single serving snacks and dry goods. ½ cup is one small muffin tin and 1 cup is 1 large one. Store in snack baggies.

13. Stackable Plastic Drawers
For storing onions and potatoes.

14. Mason Jars
For storing rice, quinoa, and other similar food items.

15. Plastic Storage Bins
Store SS, (single serving), baggies of snacks such as wheat crackers, rice cakes, corn tortilla chips, protein bars, nuts, trail mix, granola bites, cereal, popcorn, etc...

16. Desktop Magazine Holder
Store foil, saran wrap, wax paper, and other similar shaped products.

Meal Planning Strategies, Tips, & Techniques | Written By: Kristine Sinner, MS, RDN

PUTTING IT ALL TOGETHER
#HowToMealPlan

Organizing Your Groceries For Optimal Usage

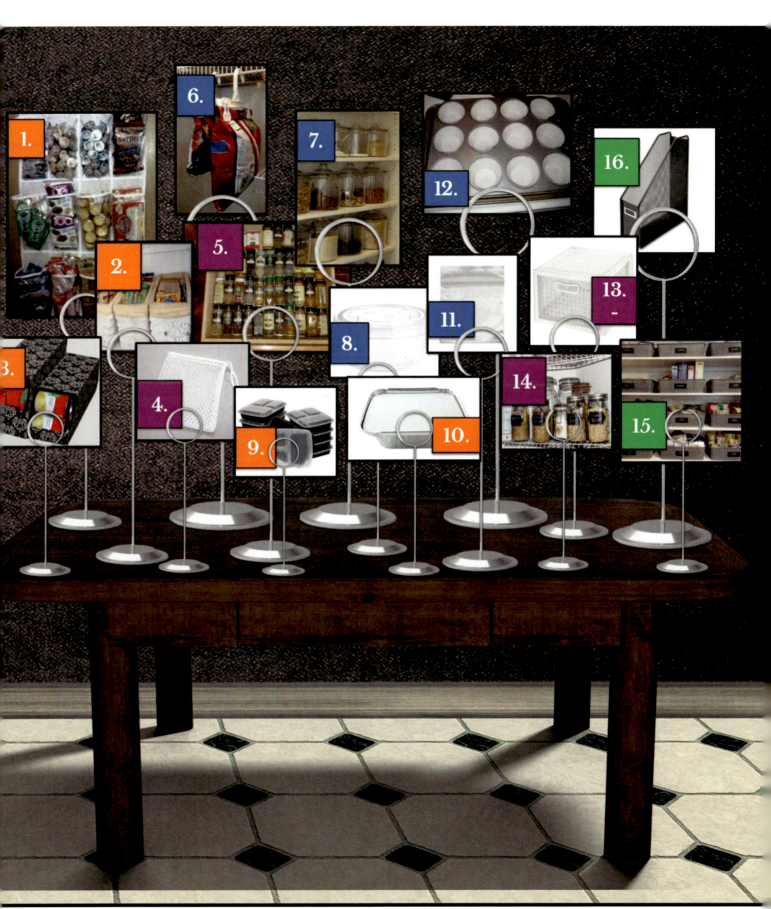

Meal Planning Strategies, Tips, & Techniques | Written By: Kristine Sinner, MS, RDN

PUTTING IT ALL TOGETHER

#HowToMealPlan

Refrigerator Single Serve Grab-n-Go Items

STORE SINGLE SERVING PORTIONS
in refrigerator drawers for easy Grab-n-Go snacks.

Remember to use snack size plastic baggies to make single servings!

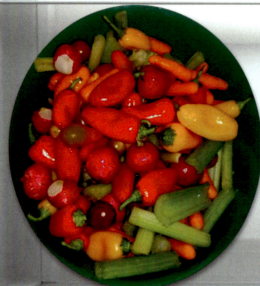

Fill a large gallon baggie of mixed portable veggies like radishes, cherry tomatoes, baby carrots, snap pea pods, green beans, celery, & mini peppers.

Take the entire bag to and from work or have it with you while running errands and eat them in the car. This is a great way to boost your veggie intake and stave off hunger between meals.

Hard Boiled Eggs	Savory Veggie dip- *Blend Non-Fat Greek yogurt and 1 Pouch of Dried Veggie Soup Mix*
Cheese-sticks, cubes, or wedges	
Deli Meat- cubed or sliced	Baggies of Apple Slices
Chocolate Milk Singles	Mixed Fruit Cups or Applesauce
Kefir Minis	Fruit - whole, single, mixed, dried
Blended Pureed Fruit Drinks	Hummus and Guac/Avocado Singles
Drinkable Mini Yogurts	Baggies of Various Vegetables
Single Serve Yogurt Cups	Pasta Spirals - Whole Grain, Veggie
Single Serve Cottage Cheese Cups	

Meal Planning Strategies, Tips, & Techniques | Written By: Kristine Sinner, MS, RDN

PUTTING IT ALL TOGETHER

Pantry Single Serve Grab-n-Go Items

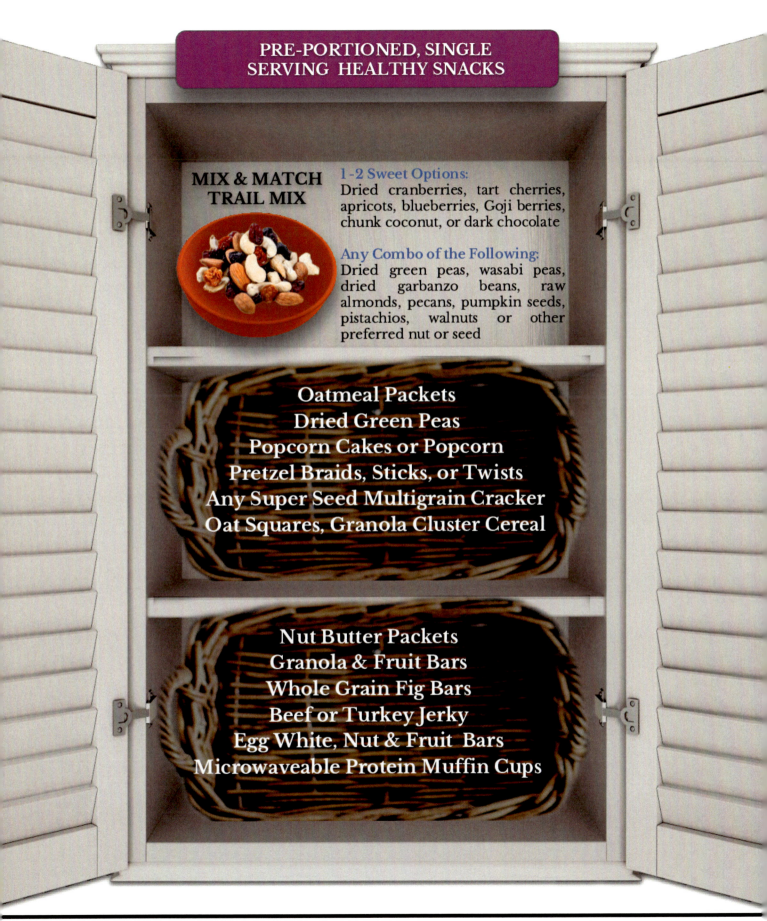

PRE-PORTIONED, SINGLE SERVING HEALTHY SNACKS

MIX & MATCH TRAIL MIX

1-2 Sweet Options:
Dried cranberries, tart cherries, apricots, blueberries, Goji berries, chunk coconut, or dark chocolate

Any Combo of the Following:
Dried green peas, wasabi peas, dried garbanzo beans, raw almonds, pecans, pumpkin seeds, pistachios, walnuts or other preferred nut or seed

Oatmeal Packets
Dried Green Peas
Popcorn Cakes or Popcorn
Pretzel Braids, Sticks, or Twists
Any Super Seed Multigrain Cracker
Oat Squares, Granola Cluster Cereal

Nut Butter Packets
Granola & Fruit Bars
Whole Grain Fig Bars
Beef or Turkey Jerky
Egg White, Nut & Fruit Bars
Microwaveable Protein Muffin Cups

APPENDIX
Meal Planning Forms & Inventories

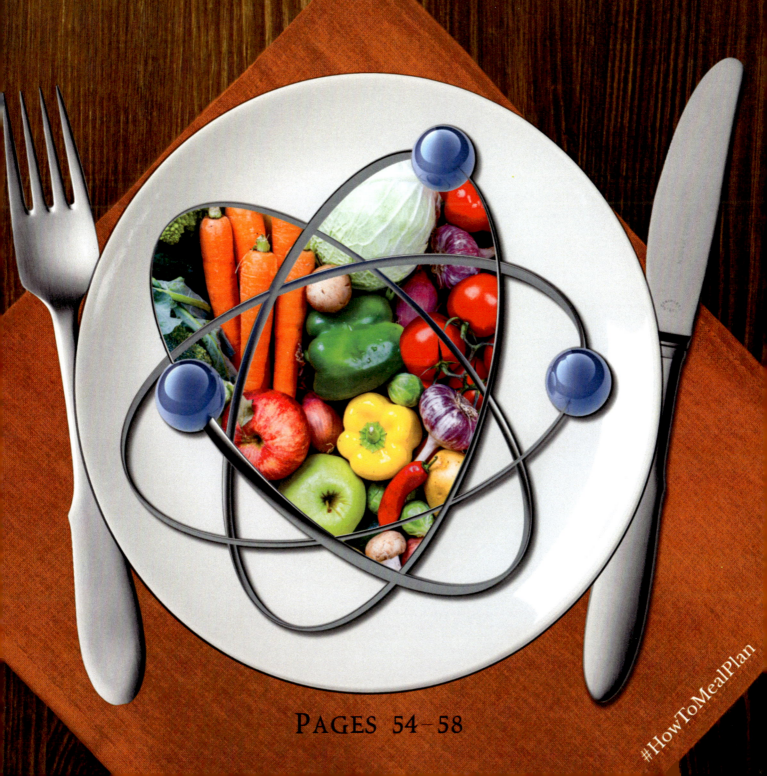

Pages 54–58

#HowToMealPlan

MY GROCERY LIST (Page 1)

Name: _____ Date: _____

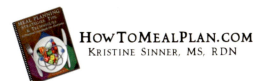

HowToMealPlan.com
Kristine Sinner, MS, RDN

Breads	Bakery	Cereals	Crackers	Cookies	Grains	Pasta	Legumes

Baking	Oils	Seasonings	Dressings	Condiments	Ethnic	Sushi	Coffee/Tea

Misc.

© 2019 by Kristine Sinner, MS, RDN. All Rights Reserved. Reprint Permission Granted For Individual Usage Only.

#HowToMealPlan

MY GROCERY LIST (Page 2)

Name: _____ Date: _____

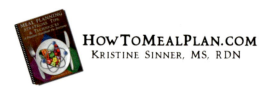

Milk	Creamer	Cheese	Yogurt	Eggs	Juice	Water	Butter

Frozen Breakfast	Frozen Vegs	Frozen Fruits	Frozen Entrees	Frozen Meats	Frozen Desserts	Household	Toiletries

Misc.

#HowToMealPlan

MASTER INVENTORY LIST

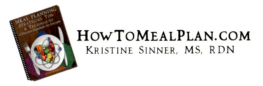

Name: _____ Date: _____

List foods currently found in your Pantry, Fridge, & Freezer

PANTRY	FRIDGE	FREEZER

© 2019 by Kristine Sinner, MS, RDN. All Rights Reserved. Reprint Permission Granted For Individual Usage Only.

#HowToMealPlan

WHAT I PLAN TO EAT THIS WEEK

Name: _____   Date: _____

HowToMealPlan.com
Kristine Sinner, MS, RDN

DAY	BREAKFAST	AM SNACK	LUNCH	PM SNACK	DINNER	HS SNACK
1						
2						
3						
4						
5						
6						
7						

© 2019 by Kristine Sinner, MS, RDN. All Rights Reserved. Reprint Permission Granted For Individual Usage Only.

#HowToMealPlan

WHAT I ATE THIS WEEK

Name: _____ Date: _____

DAY	BREAKFAST	AM SNACK	LUNCH	PM SNACK	DINNER	HS SNACK
1						
2						
3						
4						
5						
6						
7						

HowToMealPlan.com
Kristine Sinner, MS, RDN

© 2019 by Kristine Sinner, MS, RDN. All Rights Reserved. Reprint Permission Granted For Individual Usage Only.

#HowToMealPlan